O9-BHJ-867

CHICAGO PUBLIC LIBRARY

R02084 73314

Praise from the
Macular Deg

"If   ular
deg   oks
on   ove
the   as-
sior   eas,
and   ven
to   ive
the

"G   ers
pra

"   at
g   ral
vi   ok
o   rt
a   ew
e

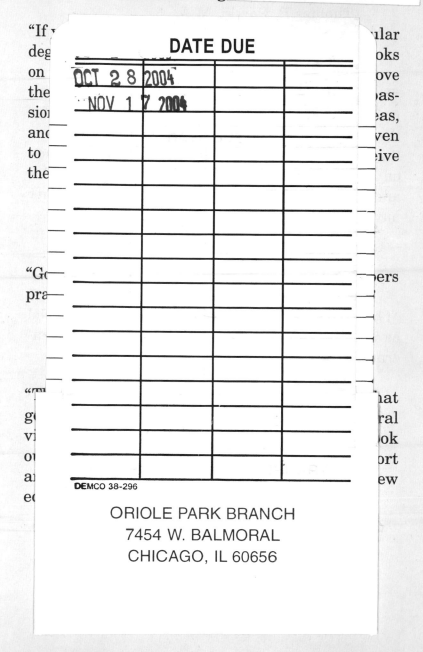

DATE DUE

OCT 2 8 2004			
NOV 1 7 2004			

DEMCO 38-296

ORIOLE PARK BRANCH
7454 W. BALMORAL
CHICAGO, IL 60656

"It is crucial that all who have an interest in macular degeneration read this book."
    —Thomas B. Perski, M.A.
      Founder and Executive Director,
      Macular Degeneration International

"This book is a feast for those of us who live with macular degeneration. It feeds our hunger for the latest medical information, and quenches our thirst for refreshing new ways of meeting each day's challenges. It's salted with inspiring tales and peppered with humor. I'm glad others won't have to wait thirty years for such a book!"
    —Fran Cutler
      Chair, National Board of Directors
      Canadian National Institute for the Blind

"This book should be read, highlighted, and used as a guide by everyone who has macular degeneration, or is at risk of developing it."
    —Robert W. Massof, Ph.D.
      Director, Lions Vision Research and
      Rehabilitation Center
      Johns Hopkins University

"An outstanding book—not only educational but inspirational. Everyone with macular degeneration, their family members, and all eye care professionals should have a copy."
—Joel A. Kraut, M.D.
Medical Director,
Vision Rehabilitation Service
Harvard Medical School

"This is the book I would want for myself if I were diagnosed with macular degeneration."
—Donald C. Fletcher, M.D.
Associate Professor of Ophthalmology
Director, Center for Vision Rehabilitation
Helen Keller Chair for Research
University of Alabama

"This is the best publication on the subject I have ever read. If you have macular degeneration or know someone who does, you must read this book! Dr. Mogk and her daughter give us straight talk and sound advice as experts and as family members."
—M. Edward Wilson, M.D.
Pierre G. Jenkins Professor and Chairman,
Department of Ophthalmology
Director, Albert Florens Storm
Eye Institute
Medical University of South Carolina

"A spectacular book—a truly important, wonderful book!"
—David R. Guyer, M.D.
Chair, Department of Ophthalmology
New York University

"An excellent book! An exciting landmark in the field—I look forward to having copies available for all of my patients."
—Robert M. Christiansen, M.D.
Director, Low Vision Services
University of Utah Medical Center

"Part personal, part analytical, all parts thoughtful, accurate, and revealing. Dr. Mogk blends her observation, knowledge, and insight to produce a wonderful guide for anyone interested in macular degeneration."
—Julian J. Nussbaum, M.D.
Professor and Chairman,
Department of Ophthalmology
Medical College of Georgia

"This is one of the rare books on low vision that I could not put down once I started reading. This book should be read by everyone with macular degeneration, as well as their families, friends, and doctors."

—Randall Jose, O.D.
Director, Houston Delta Gamma
Low Vision Center
Editor, *Understanding Low Vision*

"This special book helps your mind see 20/20, your spirit gain strength, and your eyes see all that they can."

—R. Tracy Williams, O.D.
Executive Director, Deicke Center for
Visual Rehabilitation
Wheaton, IL

"This book fills a need that is as central to visual rehabilitation as the macula is to vision itself."

—Stanley F. Wainapel, M.D., M.P.H.
Clinical Director, Rehabilitation Medicine
Albert Einstein College of Medicine, NY

"There is only one book that gives my macular degeneration patients hope: this one. Possibly only the Holy Bible can compete with it."

—Cornelis A. Verezen, B.Sc. F.A.A.O.
Director of Optometry
Ergra National Low Vision Service
The Netherlands

"Accurate and compelling—the best book on the topic by far."
—Gregory L. Goodrich, Ph.D.
Executive Board, International Society for Low Vision Rehabilitation and Research

"An excellent book! Sensitive, practical information and advice for patients and their families, friends, and physicians."
—Eleanor E. Faye, M.D.
Lighthouse International
Chair Emeritus, American Academy of Ophthalmology Vision Rehabilitation Committee

"Wonderful information for patients, relatives, and professionals."
—Aart C. Kooijman
Professor, Department of Ophthalmology
Editor, *Visual Impairment Research*
Groningen University
The Netherlands

"Lylas and Marja Mogk have written the only truly inspirational work on macular degeneration in the English language. We all need to read it."
—Philip C. Hessburg, M.D.
President, Detroit Institute of Ophthalmology

"We strongly recommend this book to our patients with AMD."
    —Gary W. Abrams, M.D.
       David Barsky Professor and
       Chair of Ophthalmology
       Kresge Eye Institute, Detroit

"Dr. Mogk's book is a beacon for those who cannot see. Her patients are very fortunate and so are all those who read it."
    —Barry W. Rovner, M.D.
       Medical Director, Geriatric Psychiatry
       Wills Eye Hospital, Philadelphia

"This is a wonderful book that provides a wealth of information. The authors are to be highly commended."
    —Gwen K. Sterns, M.D.
       Chief, Department of Ophthalmology
       Rochester General Hospital, NY

"Written with remarkable understanding and sensitivity . . . this is a special book!"
    —David K. Gieser, M.D.
       President, Wheaton Eye Clinic, IL

"I know this new edition will play a vital role in helping those with macular degeneration. This book will be a godsend."
—Lorraine H. Marchi, Ph.D.
Founder and CEO, National Association for the Visually Handicapped (NAVH)

"*Macular Degeneration* empowers people with macular degeneration to take control of their lives. I look forward to recommending this second edition to my patients, students, and colleagues."
—Mary Warren, M.S., O.T.R.
Assistant Professor of Occupational Therapy,
University of Alabama

"This book is a treasure; a must read for all who are experiencing the onset of macular degeneration, as well as for those who love them."
—Gale Watson, M.Ed., C.L.V.T.
U.S. Department of Veterans Affairs
Chair, National Board of Directors
Academy for the Certification of Vision Rehabilitation & Education Professionals

"A comprehensive, invaluable guide filled with hope and written in easily understandable language—an important book."
    —David C. Ekin, A.C.S.W., L.C.S.W.
        Executive Director, St. Louis Society for
        the Blind and Visually Impaired

"I am delighted to recommend this book for all my patients with macular degeneration, and their family members."
    —August Colenbrander, M.D.
        Chair Emeritus,
        Vision Rehabilitation Committee
        American Academy of Ophthalmology

"The pearls in this book will help everyone with macular degeneration."
    —Jeffrey T. Liegner, M.D.
        Emeritus,
        Vision Rehabilitation Committee
        American Academy of Ophthalmology

"This book belongs on the shelf of every public library."
    —Lawrence S. Evans, M.D., Ph.D.
        Director Emeritus, Low Vision Service
        Loyola University, Chicago

"Fabulous medicine—the best coverage of research and treatments, the best explanation of macular degeneration, and the best advice on the market. It's the book I choose for myself, my family, and my patients."

—Jane Barrett Kelly, M.Ed., M.D.
Associate Professor of Ophthalmology
University of California, San Francisco
Ophthalmology Editor,
Online Mendelian Inheritance
National Center of Biotechnology
National Library of Medicine

"Now everything you need to find out about AMD is available in this clear, readable book. This is indeed a contribution to making our low vision lives easier."

—Henry A. Grunwald
Former editor in chief of Time, Inc.
Author, *Twilight: Losing Sight, Gaining Insight*

MACULAR
DEGENERATION

**The Complete Guide to Saving
and Maximizing Your Sight**

**LYLAS G. MOGK, M.D.
and MARJA MOGK**

BALLANTINE BOOKS • NEW YORK

This book is not intended to replace the advice and guidance of a trained physician or optometrist, nor is it intended to encourage self-treatment of an illness or medical disease. The program in this book should be followed with approval and guidance of your physician.

A Ballantine Book
Published by The Ballantine Publishing Group

Copyright © 1999, 2003 by Lylas G. Mogk, M.D., and Marja Mogk

All rights reserved under International and
Pan-American Copyright Conventions. Published in the
United States by The Ballantine Publishing Group, a division
of Random House, Inc., New York, and simultaneously in
Canada by Random House of Canada Limited, Toronto.
This is a revised edition of a work originally published by
The Ballantine Publishing Group in 1999.

Ballantine and colophon are registered trademarks
of Random House, Inc.

www.ballantinebooks.com

Library of Congress Cataloging-in-Publication Data
is available upon request.

Text design by Holly Johnson

ISBN 0-345-45711-0

Manufactured in the United States of America

First Revised Edition: January 2003

10 9 8 7 6 5 4 3 2 1

R02084 73314

Oriole Park Branch
7454 W. Balmoral Ave.
Chicago, IL 60656

For Jack and Big Man
we love you

For
Charles R. Good

And for the many people who are striving
to meet the challenges of macular degeneration
with wisdom, grace, and humor.
You are an inspiration to us.

Contents

Contents

PART III: ADDRESSING AMD

PART IV: APPENDIXES AND INDEX

Contents

Acknowledgments

We are grateful to the many people with macular degeneration who shared their experiences with us so that others would not feel alone, to the many leaders in the macular degeneration community who have supported and inspired us, and to our colleagues in the field of low vision who have generously contributed their time and expertise. We hope that this revised edition of *Macular Degeneration: The Complete Guide* embodies the spirit of their advocacy, compassion, and dedication.

Anne Toth Riddering, M.A., O.T.R., C.L.V.T., designed the Reading Workshop in chapter 11 and the community and home visual rehabilitation program in chapter 14. She deserves credit as the coauthor of these chapters and as a wonderful colleague. Credit is also due to the outstanding staff at our visual rehabilitation center for their excellent work: Cathy Bruce, David Dahl, M.S., Shannon Brafford, C.O.A., Mary Ellen Daniel, M.A., O.T.R., C.L.V.T., and Colleen O'Donnell, M.A., O.T.R., C.L.V.T.

We would like to recognize the pivotal support of the Department of Eye Care Services of the Henry Ford Health System in Detroit, especially Paul A. Edwards, M.D., chairman, Dan

Acknowledgments

Badgley, Judi Ellis, and colleagues at Grosse Pointe Ophthalmology.

Macular Degeneration would not be the same without the contributions, suggestions, and support from leaders in the field of ophthalmology, optometry, and low vision. Many thanks to Gary W. Abrams, M.D., Ian Bailey, O.D., Robert M. Christiansen, M.D., August Colenbrander, M.D., Judith Delgado, Eleanor E. Faye, M.D., Donald C. Fletcher, M.D., David K. Gieser, M.D., Gregory L. Goodrich, Ph.D., David R. Guyer, M.D., Philip C. Hessburg, M.D., Clare M. Hood, R.N., M.A., Lea Hyvarinen, M.D., Randall Jose, O.D., Jane Barrett Kelly, M.Ed., M.D., Joel A. Kraut, M.D., Manfred Mackeben, Ph.D., Lorraine H. Marchi, Ph.D., Robert W. Massof, Ph.D., Anne Nachazel, M.D., Tomasina A. Perry, Thomas B. Perski, M.A., Greg Petersen, Dan Roberts, Bruce Rosenthal, O.D., Barry W. Rovner, M.D., Ron Schuchard, Ph.D., Karen Seidman, M.P.A., Henk L. M. Stam, B.Sc., F.A.A.O., Gwen K. Sterns, M.D., Nikolai Stevenson, Yasuo Tano, M.D., Cornelis Anton Verezen, B.Sc., F.A.A.O., Peter Verstraten, Ph.D., Meria Venhuisen, Stanley F. Wainapel, M.D., M.P.H., Mary Warren, M.S., O.T.R., Gale Watson, M.Ed., C.L.V.T., R. Tracy Williams, O.D., and M. Edward Wilson, M.D.

Our best wishes always to those who volunteered to talk with Marja about their experiences: Muriel Bleich, Geraldine Brancheau, John and Lucille Bukowicz, Eloise Craig, Lillian Danluck,

Acknowledgments

Frances Gates, Clara-Rae Genser, John Gryniewicz, Carmella Mollicone, Grethe Mumma, Sophie Plotzke, Genevieve Rentz, Geraldine Spaven, Gloria Sweeney, Sarita Thompson, Dorothy Widerstedt, Dorothy Wroten, and Catherine Yurkie. With this edition, we honor the memory of Helen Williams, Steve Sweeney, Beatrice Brandes, Helen Konkoff, Dorothy Douglass, and Edith Goldman.

We would also like to thank our family and friends for their contributions: Ed O'Malley, M.D., Wendy Kindred, Mike and Dara Pond, Chris Burmester, Lynne and Bill Mogk, Carol Gaskin, Lee Lamborn, Nancy Shalit, and Betsy Flagler.

Special thanks to Omri Aronow, chef at Rick & Ann's in Berkeley, California, for creating the gourmet greens recipes in chapter 4 especially for this edition. And special thanks to Donna Kaiser and Boffin Editorial for the appendix.

Finally, *Macular Degeneration: The Complete Guide* would not be here today without our wonderful agent, Laurie Harper of Sebastian Agency, and our dedicated editor, Allison H. Dickens. We deeply appreciate their support and advocacy on behalf of this book.

Introduction:
My Family's Story

Age-related macular degeneration (AMD) runs in my family: my father developed it in 1985 and my sister learned of her diagnosis several years ago. Since AMD runs in families, my other siblings, my children, and I may be at risk, too. This book is for all of us, across three generations, and from our family to yours. Whether you are thirty, sixty, or ninety, this book covers everything you need to know about macular degeneration.

For almost baby boomers like my sister and myself and for Gen Xers like my daughter, chapters 2 and 3 offer the latest scientific results on nutrition, natural and medical treatments, and high-tech solutions, like the eye and the chip. You'll find the stunning results of the government's landmark ARED study on vitamins and macular degeneration, the Harvard study on the importance of oils, news on natural treatments, and more. You'll also find a five-star prevention program designed to stop macular degeneration in its tracks. To help you follow the program, chapter 4 features a brand-new collection of favorite greens recipes from friends and gourmet greens designed by Omri Aronow, chef at Rick & Ann's in Berkeley, California.

If you have begun to lose vision from macular degeneration or soon may, the early chapters of this book are also for you, but parts II and III are especially so. This book is about saving sight—saving it before you lose it—but it's also about the sight that you will keep even with macular degeneration. By maximizing this sight through visual rehabilitation, you can keep the life you've built and loved. Part III provides a complete home visual rehabilitation program. Appendixes A and C provide a guide for finding professional visual rehabilitation programs in your area and low-vision products. If you still have full vision, knowing about the many elements of visual rehabilitation and using them to plan ahead is a powerful way to ensure it will always be *you* running your life and *not* macular degeneration.

For all of us—those who may lose vision, have lost vision, or know someone who has—saving sight refers to our perception of our lives. We are not all eyeball, and macular degeneration doesn't happen in a vacuum. AMD and vision loss are part and parcel of a whole life lived by a whole person. This book is also about the saving power of insight. The power of planning ahead. The power of family, friends, and physicians understanding the whole experience of vision loss. The power of people with AMD seeing themselves as so much more than a pair of eyes. Chapters 5 through 8 address the experience of macular degeneration and share the thoughts and words of some of the people with AMD whom we have had the honor to know.

NEW IN THIS EDITION

In addition to the completely revised chapters on scientific discoveries, natural and medical treatments, prevention, and greens recipes, this edition also introduces a vibrant Internet community for people with AMD and information on computers, software, and new optical aids. We've also included another tip for family and friends in chapter 7 and many more stories from people with AMD about experiencing life and living fully. You'll find a totally new chapter on driving with an expanded guide to alternatives and public transportation. We have also completely rewritten the appendixes to make them much more useful and added one for our Canadian readers, along with a new index for easy referencing. We feel honored by the enthusiastic response we received on the first edition of this book from readers and professionals in the field. This new edition is even better, and we hope it continues to be a beacon in our shared battle against AMD.

HOW IT ALL BEGAN: MY FATHER'S EXPERIENCE

My father and I are both night owls. When I was in high school I loved to stay up late, doing my homework in the kitchen while my father sat across the table, evaluating blueprints. A mechanical engineer by profession, my father was a consummate problem solver and a wonderfully patient math teacher. He was also an intensely visual person. He loved bird-watching and photography. He built a darkroom in the basement during the 1940s and developed a portfolio.

In 1985, at the age of seventy-nine, my father was diagnosed with macular degeneration in one eye. Five years later he lost the vision in his other eye, on the eve of my mother's death. My father is a naturally cheerful soul from a long line of intrepid Hungarian-Americans, but the death of his adored wife of fifty-three years, the loss of his driver's license, and his low vision were tremendous blows. He struggled with depression. I remember stopping by one afternoon, shortly after his vision had deteriorated. He was out in the yard investigating a robin's nest. "It's a shame," he said, turning to me quietly, "that Nature takes away one's sight just when we are ready to be peacefully attentive to her. I would love so much to see these birds as clearly as I once did."

Today, at ninety-seven, my father has late-stage macular degeneration, with 20/800 vision in

4

one eye and 20/500 in the other. Yet his outlook is brighter than it was several years ago. He takes long walks in the neighborhood, regularly crossing intersections of every size, shops for groceries, and uses the local buses. He bowls in a league, attends monthly senior men's club lectures, and dines out often. He particularly loves books on tape and has become an avid listener. Late at night, when we are both up at the kitchen table, he'll tell me something about the cultural revolution in China or Tony Hillerman's fiction. I really think he reads more now with his ears than he used to with his eyes.

What enables him to survive, to be happy? How did he manage to meet the enormous challenge of vision loss, combined with the other colossal losses that aging often entails, like the loss of my mother? How did he manage to turn a larger-than-life lemon into lemonade? As I approached sixty myself, with my father's light blue eyes, I found myself asking these questions and came to realize that my father had several important advantages.

First, as an engineer, he knew something about optics and how magnifiers work and could experiment with different models, finding the right one to maximize his sight. Second, his sense of himself remains remarkably unshaken. He is quite straightforward about his vision loss and doesn't hesitate to ask acquaintances to identify themselves and waiters to help with menus. He believes he is more than the sum total of his visual acuity, and he believes low vision is nothing to be embarrassed about. Finally, his daughter is an ophthalmologist, and he has access to rehabilitation services, a support group, and a full range of optical aids.

But what about the 1.5 million other Americans who have vision loss from macular degeneration and may not have these advantages? What about their friends and families? My father's experience opened my eyes to the tremendous need for accurate information, services, and support for people with AMD. In response, I opened a comprehensive visual rehabilitation program and research facility in the Department of Eye Care Services of the Henry Ford Health System in Detroit in 1997. At that time, there were no books about macular degeneration available, and we were immediately besieged with requests for information. People wanted to know the status of current research, how to prevent AMD, and how to live proactively with it. So my daughter Marja and I wrote this book to bring our program to you. It was the book I wanted for my own family then. This is the book I want for my own family now.

PART I:

Understanding AMD

CHAPTER I

What Is AMD?
A Portrait

This has become a true epidemic of
our time.

—Jerry Chader, Ph.D.
Chief Scientific Officer
The Foundation Fighting Blindness

Ten years ago, when Zelda Grant discovered she
had age-related macular degeneration, she was
astounded. "Macular what?" she said. She had
never heard of it before. Today most of us know
something about AMD, but it still comes as a
shock. "I couldn't believe it," Edina Williams told
me, "I kept thinking: I need new glasses. A new
pair will solve the problem. I still can't believe it."
Age-related macular degeneration, or AMD, is the
leading cause of adult vision loss in North America, Europe, and Australia. It affects the sight of
more adults than all of the better-known eye diseases *combined*: glaucoma, cataracts, and diabetic
retinopathy. According to the Beaver Dam Eye
Study, 18 percent of seniors aged sixty-five to
seventy-four and nearly 30 percent of seniors over

seventy-five show early evidence of the condition. One out of every twenty-five Americans over sixty-five, or nearly 1.5 million people, have already experienced significant vision loss from advanced macular degeneration, and 200,000 more Americans lose vision every year. Hundreds of thousands of people in Canada, England, Germany, and many other countries have lost vision from AMD, too. Clearly, if you have AMD you are not alone.

What Is Age-Related Macular Degeneration?

Macular degeneration dismantles central vision painlessly and silently, leaving peripheral vision intact. As a result, people with advanced macular degeneration do not feel any discomfort in their eyes and they do not appear any different to their friends and family, but their experience of the world and of their own capacities changes radically.

Because macular degeneration leaves peripheral vision intact, people with AMD can see whatever rests at the edges of their vision but cannot see clearly whatever they look at directly. They find it difficult to recognize their grandchildren's photographs, for example, but can describe the check pattern of a black-and-white tile floor. They cannot read a bus sign but can see a green leaf on the sidewalk out of the corners of their eyes. This combination of visual ability and vision loss is enormously frustrating, not the least because it takes away what we most want to see, leaving visible what appears to be less important. As Carolyn See remarked dryly in her candid article in *Modern Maturity* about living with macular degeneration, "It begins in the center of your vision and after a while you can't read or drive or recognize your relatives. They say you'll always be able to pick up a thread on the carpet. But even with full vision, picking up threads on the carpet wasn't high on my list of activities."

Why Has Macular Degeneration Suddenly Become So Common?

"Ten years ago, when I met someone on a plane en route to giving a talk and told them what I do, they would look at me kinda funny," reflected Nikolai Stevenson, president of the Association for Macular Diseases, an organization run for and by people with AMD. "With a name like 'macular degeneration,' for all they knew it was contagious. Today, though, everyone seems to know someone else with it, too: a neighbor, a friend, or a relative." Macular degeneration is no longer a stealth intruder but a known one. Why is AMD suddenly so common? Is this a new epidemic?

Doctors have actually known about macular degeneration for more than 100 years. AMD was first named by a German scientist in 1885, but the technology used to see it clearly was not developed until the 1960s. Unlike cataracts, which are visible to the naked eye, or glaucoma, which can easily be measured, macular degeneration was historically more difficult to detect, analyze, and treat. As a result, other eye conditions that were easier to understand and responded well to surgery and medication received much more attention from the medical community during the twentieth century. Macular degeneration fell to the bottom of the priority list, until now.

Are more people getting it today than ever before? Yes, but we aren't exactly sure why. On the one hand, it may be a result of our eating habits, food production methods, and the effects of more than half a century of heavy-duty industrial pollution (see chapter 3 for a discussion of the causes of macular degeneration and what you can do to minimize your risk). On the other hand, there are simply more of us today and we are living longer and healthier lives than ever before. The longer you live, the more likely you are to develop age-related macular degeneration, which doesn't usually affect people until they pass the age of fifty and increases exponentially every decade thereafter (hence the prefix *age-related*).

It's also true that many of our parents or grandparents may have had macular degeneration, but we didn't recognize their vision loss as a disease. We saw it simply as a sign of growing old. I remember my own grandmother stooped over in the garden wearing her black dress and black shoes, with her gray hair tucked in a bun. It was 1947 and she was only sixty-nine, but we thought she was very, very, very old. We also knew she couldn't see well, but no one had a special name for that. Today sixty-nine is looking pretty young. The folks in their late sixties I see at our visual rehabilitation program in Michigan come in wearing very spiffy outfits and have a good fifteen to thirty more good years of reading, entertaining, traveling, and sports ahead of them. Some of them aren't even retired. In fact, sometimes I see ninety-year-olds who fit that description. If I suggested that they wear black, put their hair in a bun, and act old like my grandma was, they'd probably slug me. Seniors today aren't old the way they used to be, and they aren't willing to pass off age-related macular degeneration as something that "just happens" when you're "old," nor should they.

Macular Degeneration Gains Attention

In the last ten years, macular degeneration has become a major health issue. The National Eye Institute (NEI), a division of the National Institutes of Health, has made AMD its number-one priority, and Medicare has approved national coverage for visual rehabilitation for people with vision loss. Studies are underway at major research centers across the country to discover the genetic components of AMD and its environmental causes and to find a cure. Many new surgeries and treatments are on the horizon. Chapter 2, "Medical Treatments, Research, and New Discoveries," outlines all of the exciting new developments in the field. For the latest research updates, see the resources listed in appendix E. We now know for sure that nutrition can help prevent the disease: what you eat does make a difference. See chapter 3, "Genes, Greens, and Oils: The Causes, Prevention, and Natural Treatment of AMD," for details and diet recommendations. Macular degeneration is complicated, and so far there is no single easy answer—but we do have some answers and we have a very strong hope that many more are soon to come.

Macular Degeneration Isn't Just About Your Eyes

Most people say they'd rather lose a limb than an eye, and national surveys tend to place vision loss among the most feared afflictions, along with Alzheimer's. Why? Because eyesight affects every aspect of life: mobility, physical activity, communication, appearance, perception, self-esteem, and psychological health. Macular degeneration is not just about how much you can or cannot see. It's about your whole life: how you cope with change, your view of the future, and your capacity to enjoy the present. And macular degeneration is tailor-made to push every button we have. It can raise feelings of grief, helplessness, depression, fear, anxiety, and anger. Part II of this book addresses these experiences and how you can live fully with AMD, but first we have to really understand the condition itself. As Zelda put it, "Macular what?" What is this macular degeneration really?

AGE-RELATED MACULAR DEGENERATION EXPLAINED

Our Eyes Are Like Little Cameras

You have probably heard this analogy before: Our eyes are like little cameras. Just as light enters the camera through the shutter, is focused

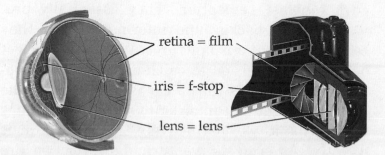

retina = film

iris = f-stop

lens = lens

The human eye is like a camera. While the film is simply a strip in the back of the camera, the retina lines the entire inside of the eyeball.

by the lens, and falls on the film, so light enters our eye through the pupil, is focused by the lens, and falls on the retina at the back of our eye. The retina is like camera film. Its thin tissue forms the inner lining of the eye, picking up light and converting it into nerve signals. The retina sends those signals through the optic nerve to the brain, which "develops" them into the images we actually see, just as film is developed into photographs.

The Macula: Center of the Retina

The retina has two types of photoreceptor cells that convert light into electrical messages for the optic nerve to transmit: rod cells and cone cells, so named for their shapes. There are many more rods than cones throughout the retina, especially at the edges, where rods outnumber cones twenty to one. Rod cells are responsible for light-and-dark contrast perception. They essentially provide us with background information, but they cannot transmit crisp pictures. We use the rods of our peripheral vision to catch a glimpse of something. They tell us that a car is coming from the far left or right, but in order to see the car clearly or describe it, we instinctively turn to look at it directly. As soon as we turn, however, we are no longer primarily using our rod cells to see but our cone cells. Cones are concentrated in the center of the retina—called the macula—and are re-

sponsible for central vision, color perception, and
sharp images (acute vision). The capacity of cones
to distinguish detail is one hundred times greater
than that of rods. We need them to tell the difference between forest green and black and to
see precise detail, such as the features of a face,
the lace pattern on a tablecloth, and the letters on
this page. The macula is therefore both the geographic center of the retina and the focal center of
our vision. The fovea is the very center of the
macula. It is also the only area of the retina that
has only cone cells. For all its power, though, the
macula is very small; it measures about a quarter

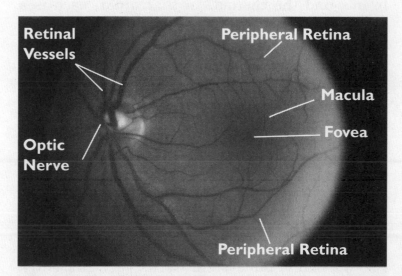

**Photograph of the inside of a normal eye. This is
what doctors see when they look into your eye.**

inch in diameter and is tissue paper thin. But the macula is truly a mouse that roars. This tiny area is responsible for so much of what we see.

Macular Degeneration: The Key Players

In macular degeneration, rod and cone cells of the macula begin to die, reducing the number of cells able to transmit visual signals to the brain. Macular degeneration, however, is not a condition of these cells alone but also of the underlying tissue that supports them and keeps them healthy. In addition to the rods and cones, there are three more key players in macular degeneration: the retinal pigment epithelium (RPE), Bruch's membrane, and the choroid. In that order, each is a layer of tissue that lies beneath the retina, like layers of a club sandwich or, more accurately, stations on a delivery line. Taken together, they form a kind of conveyor belt for nutrition and waste management, constantly supplying the macula with oxygen-laden meals and whisking away waste. The large blood vessels of the choroid truck materials in and out through the bloodstream. Bruch's membrane acts as a security gate between these blood vessels and the delicate RPE, and the RPE delivers oxygen and receives waste directly from the rod and cone cells in the macula.

Normally, the system works very efficiently. But if there's a jam somewhere, the oxygen meal shipments and the waste removals back up, clogging the pickup and drop-off stations until they eventually shut down. The choroid, Bruch's membrane, and the RPE become disabled and can no longer do their jobs. When they fail, the rod and cone cells lack the massive amounts of oxygen they need to stay alive and cannot clear away the waste products they produce. Dying of oxygen deprivation and clogged with refuse, rods and cones become unable to send signals through the optic nerve to the brain—they are no longer able to see. This is what happens with macular degeneration.

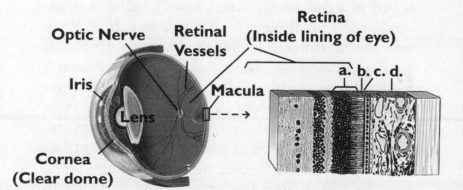

Eye showing cross section of the "conveyor belt." a. cones and rods, b. retinal pigment epithelium (RPE), c. Bruch's membrane, d. choroid.

TWO TYPES OF AMD: DRY AND WET

There are two types of macular degeneration, commonly called dry and wet. All cases are thought to start with the dry form. Between 10 and 15 percent of the people who show signs of dry macular degeneration eventually develop the wet form.

Dry AMD

Although there is only one kind of dry AMD, you may hear it called atrophic, geographic atrophy, or nonexudative macular degeneration. *Atrophic* or *atrophy* refers to a declining, weakening, or wasting away. We often use the word to talk about muscles that haven't been used in a great while and lose their strength as a result. We can exercise our muscles and regain strength, but unlike our muscles, atrophy in our macula isn't currently reversible. This is because the macula atrophies from a lack of oxygen, not a lack of use. And, as we know, any part of our body that suffers a prolonged lack of oxygen usually sustains permanent damage. *Geographic atrophy* of the macula means atrophy concentrated in one contiguous area of the macula. *Nonexudative* means not exuding, or not discharging: there is no blood leakage in the macula, contributing to the malfunctioning of the conveyor belt system.

HARD AND SOFT DRUSEN

Dry AMD is usually signaled by the presence in the macula of small pale spots called *drusen*. There are two type of drusen: less harmful hard drusen and more ominous soft drusen. Hard drusen are small, round, sharply defined light yellow deposits of lipid (a fatty compound) and calcium that accumulate on Bruch's membrane. They are quite common with age, appearing in most older eyes like age spots appear on skin, and are not necessarily thought to indicate macular degeneration. Soft drusen can be nearly twice the size of hard drusen, with indistinct margins and varying sizes and shapes. While soft drusen can be seen in older eyes that don't develop full-blown AMD, they have been considered an early indicator of the condition, perhaps because they are the first feature of AMD that we can detect in an affected eye. Recently, however, researchers have suggested that by the time we can see soft drusen in an eye, macular degeneration may already be advanced.

Soft drusen are thought to plug up the conveyor belt system in dry macular degeneration. Some researchers also believe that soft drusen are responsible for wet macular degeneration because they may weaken Bruch's membrane or because they may trigger the proliferation of abnormal blood vessels. Other researchers disagree, arguing that soft drusen occur because Bruch's membrane has already been weakened for some other reason. In any case, soft drusen signal to us that the conveyor belt support system for the macula is malfunctioning and Bruch's membrane is weak, which may allow abnormal blood vessels from the choroid to creep through.

FOCAL HYPERPIGMENTATION

Like both hard and soft drusen, focal hyperpigmentation is a signal of possible early macular degeneration that your ophthalmologist can see during a standard dilated eye exam with no special testing. *Focal hyperpigmentation* means the appearance of darkish irregular specks in the macula. These specks are caused by pigment cells that clump up over time, although we aren't sure exactly why they do. Although the retina is transparent, it appears to us as reddish-orange because the underlying RPE and choroid give it color. The light yellow color of drusen and the darkish pigment flecks of focal hyperpigmentation show up against this red-orange glow. Macular degeneration is a condition of gradual deterioration and these changes indicate, at the very least, that the process is beginning.

Wet AMD

Wet AMD is called wet because it is characterized by new abnormal leaky blood vessels that grow underneath the retina in the choroid. You may also hear wet AMD called subretinal net, subretinal neovascularization (SRNV), or choroidal neovascularization (CNV). *Subretinal* means underneath the retina or underneath the RPE, and *neovascularization* simply means new vessels. Wet AMD may also be referred to as exudative degeneration. *Exudative* means seeping or bleeding, referring to these abnormal blood vessels. We don't know why these abnormal blood vessels grow. They grow from the choroid through

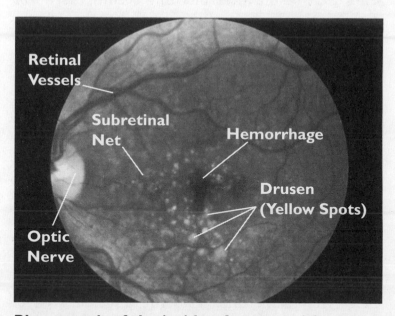

Photograph of the inside of an eye with wet AMD, showing drusen, hemorrhage, and subretinal net.

Bruch's membrane, which is not supposed to allow such a thing, and collect under the RPE like tree roots under a sidewalk.

The walls of these vessels are weak and they tend to leak clear fluid (like the fluid that accumulates when something swells up in the body) and blood. These liquids seep through the surrounding tissue, flooding the cone cells of the macula and either suffocating them or triggering changes that result in their death. Very late–stage wet macular degeneration is sometimes called disciform degeneration. Although this refers to the disc-shaped scars that result after bleeding occurs, *disciform degeneration* is generally used to simply refer to extensive or late-stage degeneration.

If these vessels leak enough, they may lift the RPE away from Bruch's membrane, creating a sort of blister between the two layers that permanently destroys the conveyor belt system in that particular area. This condition is called a serous pigment epithelial detachment, or PED. A PED is sometimes referred to in patient information pamphlets as a third type of macular degeneration, but it is a possible development in wet macular degeneration.

Your ophthalmologist may be able to detect the presence of these abnormal blood vessels, because they sometimes give the affected area of your retina a muted gray-green color. But to define the precise size and shape of these vessels, an angiogram is necessary. This is a photograph of your eye taken with a special camera that can detect dye in blood vessels. Having an angiogram involves having dye injected into your arm. This dye travels throughout your bloodstream, making all of your blood, including the blood in those abnormal vessels, glow for the camera. Chapter 2 provides a more detailed explanation of both kinds of angiograms commonly used, as well as treatments for macular degeneration.

WHEN AMD APPEARS

Macular degeneration may catch you off-guard if you don't see your eye doctor for a checkup every two years. Early signs of AMD are easily detectable to your doctor before you lose any vision. However, since AMD progresses painlessly and silently and our eyes are designed to compensate for each other, some folks lose vision from macular degeneration without realizing that they have.

Buddy Burmester's experience, for example, is common. He found over time that there wasn't enough light in the kitchen to read the paper, so he turned on another one or sat out in the sun, without really noticing his own adjustment. It wasn't until street signs became difficult to see at dusk that he thought he might need new glasses. Like Zelda, he was utterly shocked to discover that his eyesight in his right eye was 20/200, at the level of legal blindness, while his left eye was

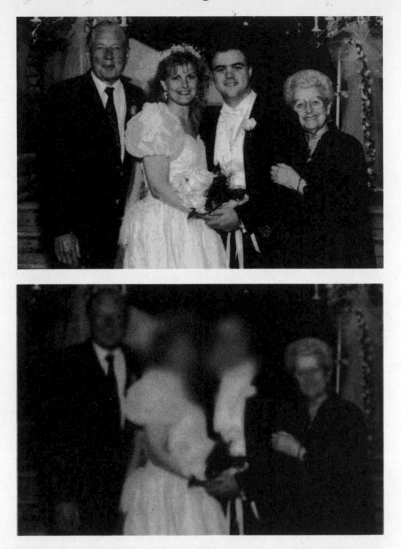

Macular degeneration damages or destroys central vision but doesn't affect the rest of the visual field. When the center is gone, the best remaining vision is at the edges of the lost central field. This example shows mild AMD.

holding its own at 20/50. How could he lose this much vision without knowing it? Our brain is hardwired to ignore visual problems by ignoring the eye that produces them and relying on the other one, especially in the case of gradual vision loss. Buddy's brain fooled him by looking through his better eye.

If you have been told that you have early-stage macular degeneration, you should monitor your vision by using an Amsler grid (see chapter 2). This is important because many of the medical treatments we have target wet macular degeneration and require immediate treatment when blood vessels are forming under the macula. Since blood vessel growth in the macula is painless, you may not know it has happened unless you monitor your vision. In any case, see your eye doctor every two years and if you ever notice changes in your vision call him or her immediately.

Your Risk of Developing Macular Degeneration

If you have some soft drusen, which is usually considered a sign of early-onset AMD, you may never develop late-stage macular degeneration and significant vision loss. The risk, however, increases with age and with other factors, like eye color, family background, a history of smoking, and diet. See chapter 3 for a longer discussion of all of these risk factors and what you can do to reduce them. Unfortunately, there are no reliable risk statistics for dry AMD, which means that we cannot really predict how fast your dry macular degeneration may progress, whether you will get it in both eyes, or what amount of vision you may lose. What remains clear, however, is that everyone's risk of macular degeneration increases with age. If you are fifty-five, for example, your chance of having early signs of macular degeneration is about 14 percent and your chance of having full-blown macular degeneration (either wet or dry) is about one-half percent. By the time you are over seventy-five, however, these figures jump to 30 percent and 7 percent, respectively.

Your Risk of Developing Wet AMD in a Second Eye

Researchers have focused most of their efforts on wet macular degeneration, since wet macular degeneration causes vision loss more quickly and extensively than the dry form. We do not have accurate statistics on the risk of developing wet macular degeneration to start with, but if you have it in one eye already, the Macular Photocoagulation Study isolated four risk factors for developing AMD in your second eye:

1. Five or more drusen in your second eye

2. More than one druse larger than .064 millimeters

3. Focal hyperpigmentation (little areas of pigment clumping in the RPE)

4. High blood pressure

According to this study, your risk of developing wet macular degeneration in your second eye within five years of the first eye is as follows: 7 percent with no risk factors, 25 percent with one risk factor, 44 percent with two risk factors, 53 percent with three risk factors, and 87 percent with four risk factors. There is a possible fifth risk factor. A recent study found that if you have PED in your first eye, your risk of losing vision in your second eye is greater. However, none of these figures and facts tell us how much vision you may lose. There's still a lot we're figuring out, because macular degeneration isn't very predictable. It varies greatly from one person to another.

Macular Degeneration Isn't Predictable

Some people have dry macular degeneration for years and never develop the wet form, while others develop the wet form right away. Some people who have had macular degeneration for years are still driving their cars and reading standard print; others who have had it for months have lost much more of their central vision. Macular degeneration just isn't predictable. We don't know yet why there are such great differences between people's experiences. We may find that there are several distinct types of macular degeneration— some genetic, some mild, some aggressive—that we haven't yet distinguished from one another. There are many researchers at work right now answering this question.

LATE-STAGE AMD

Given that we can't predict how macular degeneration may affect any particular person, what is the worst-case scenario? How bad does it get? What exactly does "developing vision loss" mean anyway? The phrase sounds like a polite euphemism, largely because we have an impoverished vocabulary for talking about visual impairment. Until very recently, our options were to talk about having normal vision or being blind, with the confusing third term *legal blindness* in the mix (see chapter 5 for a description of the unique patterns of vision that macular degeneration causes).

AMD Affects Only the Macula, Not the Whole Retina

Macular degeneration is by definition a condition that affects only the macula—*not* the entire retina. It is a failure of the tissue that supports the macula to keep it clear of waste and supplied with adequate oxygen. This failure occurs in the macula alone because it is the only place in the retina with a very high concentration of cone cells packed into a very tiny area and cone cells turn out to be very demanding. They consume enormous quantities of oxygen and produce enormous quantities of oxygenated waste. In fact, the macula uses more oxygen for its size than any other area of the body. The rest of the retina has a higher concentration of rod cells that are less demanding and are distributed over a larger area so there's more support tissue available for each cell. It might help to think of the macula as a busy little island in the middle of a big, calm retina rod lake: the macula has its own soil, its own root system, and its own drama of health and survival.

Total Blindness

The good news is that no one goes totally blind from macular degeneration. If you have AMD and no other eye condition, you will always have some peripheral vision. This sight is yours to keep, a saving grace that will enable you to maintain a level of independence and to enjoy activities that require some vision. But how can we be so sure? After all, we admittedly don't know as much as we'd like to about macular degeneration and its causes. And if physicians don't know exactly what triggers the development of soft drusen or the proliferation of abnormal blood vessels in the macula, then how can they guarantee that total blindness from macular degeneration isn't a possibility? The answer is that this guarantee is built into the anatomy of your eye. As the preceding section explains, macular degeneration by definition is a degeneration of the *macula*—not the entire retina. The cells outside the macula that provide your peripheral vision, and their supporting tissue, remain unaffected by macular degeneration.

Having said this so emphatically, there is one unusual exception. In very rare cases the bleeding from abnormal blood vessels in the macula from wet AMD is so profuse that it floods the entire retina. When this happens, peripheral vision may also be reduced, but this is extremely rare. Those with other advanced eye conditions in addition to macular degeneration, such as glaucoma, may also lose peripheral vision. For this reason, it's critical to see your eye doctor regularly and follow all prescribed treatment plans. Under no circumstances, however, does anyone experience total darkness as a result of macular degeneration alone.

The Fear of Total Blindness

Since AMD is a degenerative condition, it can be doubly frustrating because it can subject those who have it to comparisons with the past and worrying conjectures on the future. "Last year I could read the newspaper; this year I cannot." "Tomorrow the saltshaker will disappear—and who knows what else with it." It's enough to drive even the most stalwart personality nuts and lead to a very real fear of total blindness. The good news is that except in the very rarest cases of wet AMD, macular degeneration will not affect your peripheral vision, so you will not become blind in the way that we usually think of that word. The problem is that peripheral vision is not very precise, which raises the question: "How much more central vision can I lose and still really see?" This is the question that many patients would like to throw at their doctors' assurances that they are not at risk of blindness. "What, in other words, is the practical difference between what you are calling blindness and what I'm seeing or, more precisely, what I'm not seeing?"

The practical difference is enormous, especially if you work to enhance your remaining eyesight through visual rehabilitation. Vision that is 20/400, while not close to 20/20, is a great deal more sight than what we commonly call blindness. My ninety-seven-year-old father has 20/500 vision in his better eye from macular degeneration. He bowls in a league, writes his own checks, and dines out regularly. He once took a bus up to the frame shop, had his favorite photograph enlarged, gave instructions for cropping it, and selected a matching silver frame. And then he walked home. That's a lot more than he could do if he truly couldn't see anything at all.

OUR VOCABULARY OF VISION

Blind is a loaded word in our culture. We have all kinds of images of blindness and reactions to the word that aren't necessarily realistic or even rational, and we often wind up miscommunicating when we use it. To the fully sighted, *blind* usually means not being able to see anything at all, but most people who identify as blind have some usable vision. Then there's *legally blind*, which is an entirely different bird, and *low vision*, which is a third bird—and then there's the ubiquitous *20/20*. Sorting out what all these terms means helps us find a language to explain our experience of vision.

20/20

We often think of 20/20 vision as perfect sight. We say "hindsight is twenty-twenty" or we name a truth-finding television program *20/20*. The truth is that 20/20 vision is not perfect vision but *standard vision*, vision that is considered average normal (some people have better than 20/20 vision). The first 20 represents you standing twenty feet away from an object. The second figure, in this case also a 20, represents how far away from the object a person with standard normal eyes could stand and still see it in the same amount of detail as you do. In other words, if your vision is 20/60, it means that what you can see from a distance of 20 feet the average person with normal eyes can see from a distance of 60 feet. We can take Buddy Burmester as an example. When he discovered that the vision in his right eye was 20/200, it meant that he could see the same level of detail from 20 feet away that his wife or daughter could see from 200 feet away.

This figure, however, doesn't give a complete picture of the quality of your vision. There are a whole host of other variables that go into measuring visual acuity that the figures 20/60 and 20/200 don't represent. For example, 20/60 doesn't measure visual ability in varying weather or lighting conditions and it doesn't measure color perception or contrast sensitivity. The only other measure that has gained as widespread a use as the 20/20 measure is the field measure. The average normal eye has a visual field of roughly 170 degrees, or a little less than a half circle. This means that when you look straight ahead and stretch out your arms to either side, you can see from the tip of one hand to the tip of the other out of the corners of your eyes. This is the peripheral vision that the vast majority of people with macular degeneration keep.

Vision Exists on a Continuum

Using the 20/20 measure as our sole vocabulary for vision is misleading because it suggests to us that seeing is an all-or-nothing proposition, rather than a process. We talk about whether we have 20/20 vision or not. We measure our sight based on a number we get from the optometrist's or ophthalmologist's office rather than on what we can accomplish with our eyes. We fall into thinking that there are two categories of people in the world: those who can see and those who can't, or the normal and the blind. But vision exists on a continuum, like hearing or feeling pain. Whenever we experience pain we are aware of its quality and intensity. Doctors often ask, "On a scale of one to ten, how much back pain do you feel?" We think of hearing on a relative scale, too. Music that one person experiences as too loud another may experience as not loud enough. When people say they are "hard of hearing" we accept that they have some amount of hearing loss, but we aren't sure how much—it depends upon the individual. This variation is true of vision, too.

Lorraine Marchi, a pioneer advocate in the field of low vision and the founder of the National Association for the Visually Handicapped (NAVH), coined the term *hard of seeing* as a more accurate description for most types of vision loss than the word *blind* connotes. Many blind people perceive some light, and may recognize light sources or even see some hand motion. People with low vision see much more than hand motion but less than about 20/60. That's a very big range. We need to get used to thinking about *low vision*, rather than *perfect vision* versus *blindness*. *Low vision* includes a wide range of visual ability that is less than 20/20 but more than blind. Simply, as Mrs. Marchi says, it's "hard of seeing."

Legal Blindness

Legal blindness does not mean total blindness. The federal government created the term *legal blindness* during the Great Depression as a designation for people whose vision was low enough that they would have trouble finding employment and needed special relief money (the original term was *economic blindness*). The government simply used the big *E* on the eye chart: if you couldn't see the big *E*, you were legally blind. This translates into 20/200 sight in your best eye or less with glasses, or a visual field of 20 degrees or less. *Legal blindness* is an anachronistic term, even though we still use it, because it was determined before the advent of visual aids and computer software. Today many people who are legally blind have jobs that require sight and many do not consider themselves blind. In fact, more than 85 percent of the legally blind in this country have some functional vision; only 15 percent are completely blind. The biggest significance of *legal blindness* today is still what it was seventy years ago: if you qualify you are entitled to tax benefits and access to programs at your state commission for the blind (see appendixes A and D; Canadians see appendix F).

Low Vision

Using *low vision* avoids the limitations of other terms like *20/20, blind,* and *legally blind.* And the term approximates what is actually going on, which is the presence of vision with impairment. It's a term we can use to talk about the varieties of vision that people experience, rather than continually struggling with the twin poles of perfect vision and total blindness. The term covers such a wide range of visual abilities that various health, government, and private organizations define it slightly differently. Insurance reimbursement policies and state regulations differ quite a bit. For example, many states require 20/40 vision or better for an unrestricted driver's license, while others allow people with vision of 20/100 to drive (see chapter 13). Medicare recognizes 20/70 or less as qualifying for visual rehabilitation services, while many state programs require 20/200 or less (see chapter 9). The NEI recommends that low vision be defined in terms of ability rather than by a particular acuity on the 20/20 scale. We ought to be asking, in other words, whether or not someone can read a newspaper or a label or recognize a friend on the street when we seek to define that person's vision.

GLAUCOMA, CATARACTS, AND MACULAR DEGENERATION

Finally, people often ask me if glaucoma, cataracts, or diabetic retinopathy aggravates macular

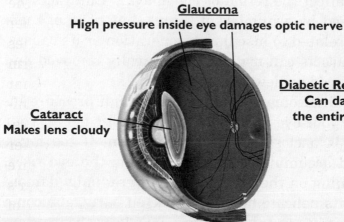

Glaucoma
High pressure inside eye damages optic nerve

Diabetic Retinopathy
Can damage
the entire retina

Cataract
Makes lens cloudy

Glaucoma, cataracts, and diabetic retinopathy affect the eye differently from AMD. They are not related conditions.

degeneration or if macular degeneration aggravates any of them. The answer is no. AMD is not directly related to any other disease or eye condition to our knowledge. There is some evidence that cataract *surgery* might affect macular degeneration. Chapter 2 discusses this possible relationship in greater detail. To understand why glaucoma, cataracts, diabetic retinopathy, and macular degeneration are unrelated, it may help to return to our original picture of the eye and clarify how each of these conditions causes vision loss.

Cataracts occur when the lens on the front of your eyes clouds up. This opacity prevents images and light from entering your eye, sort of the same way sheer curtains block the view through a window. Unlike macular degeneration, cataracts do not affect the retina or the macula. Cataracts are caused by a number of things, but none of them are related to macular degeneration or its causes. Cataracts can usually be surgically removed and replaced by new lenses.

Glaucoma is a condition of high pressure inside your eye that damages your optic nerve. Your eye is a closed, fluid-filled system. If too much fluid accumulates, pressure inside the eye rises, pushing on the optic nerve and gradually damaging its delicate fibers. If detected early, glaucoma is easily treatable in most people with prescription eyedrops, laser, or surgery. If untreated or uncontrolled, glaucoma can cause peripheral vision loss and eventually complete blindness.

Diabetic retinopathy is a condition caused by diabetes in which the retina may become swollen and abnormal blood vessels may develop on the surface of the retina. These vessels can bleed or constrict and cause retinal detachment. Diabetic retinopathy can affect the entire retina, resulting in different degrees of vision loss. It is treatable with laser in most people if identified early enough. *You cannot get diabetic retinopathy if you do not have diabetes.* People with diabetes have a higher incidence of glaucoma and cataracts but not of macular degeneration.

CHAPTER 2

Medical Treatments, Research, and New Discoveries

We are at the brink of understanding
the basic mechanisms of AMD. We
are truly in an exciting time.
—Hans E. Grossniklaus, M.D.
Addressing the American Academy of
Ophthalmology
November 2001

History tells us that surgical
sophistication will solve this problem,
as it has for so many others.
—Yasuo Tano, M.D.
Gertrude Payton Award Lecture, 2001

Macular degeneration is now one of the hottest research topics in ophthalmology. With so many studies underway, the research landscape can be bewildering. This chapter is designed to give you a solid overview of current treatments, new discoveries, and ongoing studies, so that you'll have a clear picture of your options and what to expect in the near future and can easily evaluate new research updates as you hear about them. For the very latest updates, visit the following Web sites: the NEI at www.nei.nih.gov, the Foundation Fighting Blindness at www.blindness.org, MD Partnership at www.amd.org, and MD Support at www.mdsupport.org. If you do not use computers, you can join one or more of the macular degeneration organizations listed in appendix A and receive their large-print newsletters, which provide research updates.

WHERE WE ARE AND WHERE WE'RE GOING

There are three treatments for macular degeneration that have been proven effective: the traditional form of laser called laser photocoagulation, an exciting new form of laser called photodynamic therapy, or PDT, which uses the drug Visudyne, and vitamin supplements. Both types of laser can treat only wet macular degeneration and are effective in delaying additional vision loss in 70 percent of the people who receive treatment. So what exactly is laser? What is PDT and what makes it different from traditional laser? Are they for you? Why do we hear so many reports of research breakthroughs and new treatments in the media, but only two forms of laser are available? What kinds of research are ongoing right now? How can you participate? What discoveries should we expect in the near future? These are all questions we aim to answer in this chapter. For more information on vitamin supplements and their importance in treating macular degeneration, see chapter 3, "Genes, Greens, and Oils: The Causes, Prevention, and Natural Treatment of AMD."

Ten years ago, at a national ophthalmology meeting, every famous retinal specialist I could think of stood onstage. They hung their heads together and said, "We don't have anything really effective to offer for macular degeneration." Everyone in the room felt their sadness. If you've spent your whole life believing that you can save others' sight with your medical skills, meeting macular degeneration means that you've met your match. As one of my colleagues confessed recently, "We feel absolutely horrible that we can't offer anything that will really cure macular degeneration. And then we have to tell someone the bad news. It's an awful feeling." Today we still don't have treatments for everyone with macular degeneration and we don't have any 100 percent effective treatment, but we are much closer to that dream today than we were just a decade ago. Today every national meeting is packed with ophthalmologists eager for news and research results and there's lots to share. But laser has prolonged the central vision of thousands of people over the years and is still the treatment of choice. So we'll start the story there.

LASER

Whether you're having the traditional form of laser (laser photocoagulation) or PDT (photodynamic therapy), you're still having laser. *Laser* is actually an acronym. It stands for **L**ight **A**mplification by **S**timulated **E**mission of **R**adiation. The name is confusing because it sounds like laser is an X ray, but as we know from movies, laser is an extremely fine beam of radiated light. Many patient brochures refer to "laser surgery," while others call it "laser treatment," but it's the same procedure either way. Laser for macular degeneration works on the abnormal blood vessels that develop with wet macular degeneration. Your ophthalmologist cauterizes each leaky blood vessel underneath the macula with laser, in hopes of preventing the vessel from leaking any further. The procedure affects only the macula and the tissue underneath, leaving other areas of your eye untouched.

As a treatment option, laser has several big advantages. First, it is quick, because the radiation beam takes only a fraction of a second to do its job. Also, laser is usually painless, because your retina has no pain nerve endings, only visual nerve endings. And since the area of the macula that is treated has lost some of its ability to see, the laser's bright light is not usually irritating. Extensive laser treatment in a short period of time may cause discomfort and local anesthesia may be given, but most people with macular degeneration tolerate laser quite easily. Finally, laser is not incapacitating. The procedure is done in your ophthalmologist's office and requires no eye patches or special medicine regimen. You should be able to walk out minutes later and continue your daily routine.

The First Step: Early Detection

Early detection of wet macular degeneration is necessary for laser to be effective. One of the great drawbacks of laser is that it cannot restore lost vision. When abnormal blood vessels grow and leak, they swamp the photoreceptor cells in the macula with blood, causing them to die. Laser can stop a particular blood vessel from leaking further, but it cannot revive these dead cones. It's essential to detect these renegade vessels and laser them before they do too much damage, rather than afterward. In some cases, though, people do experience slightly improved vision from laser when the blood pooling in their maculas drains away. The best way to detect these leaky blood vessels early is to monitor your vision regularly with an Amsler grid.

Early Detection: Using the Amsler Grid

Most patient brochures about AMD reprint the Amsler grid, so you may have seen it before. By looking at the Amsler grid with each eye separately and noticing whether the appearance of the grid lines has changed, you may be able to tell whether or not new blood vessels are developing in your macula. Waviness in the lines, dark spots on the grid, and choppiness are all typical distortions caused by a network of blood vessels under the retina. If they are detected early enough, your doctor may be able to treat these blood vessels with laser.

Because wet macular degeneration may develop from the dry form, most ophthalmologists give the Amsler grid to all of their macular degeneration patients, even though laser is only useful for wet AMD. Many brochures suggest checking your vision daily. If you are experiencing early-onset wet macular degeneration, this is very important. But checking your vision daily is not necessary for many people, particularly those with very advanced dry macular degeneration. If you have early to moderate dry AMD, checking weekly may be sufficient. Talk with your doctor about the Amsler grid and ask his or her advice on how often you should check your eyesight. If you do not have AMD, you should see an eye doctor every two years for a checkup.

HOW TO USE THE AMSLER GRID

1. Use the same lighting and put on your regular reading glasses each time.

2. Cover your right eye.

3. Hold the grid at your usual reading distance. Look only at the dot in the center of the grid.

4. If any lines around the dot are wavy, choppy, or distorted or if a dark spot appears on the grid, tell your ophthalmologist immediately.

5. Cover your left eye and repeat the same steps.

Side Effects of the Amsler Grid

Unfortunately, widespread use of the Amsler grid has caused three unintended "side effects." The first side effect is that some people feel terribly guilty once they discover their vision loss and find that there is such a thing as an Amsler grid. "Why didn't I detect my vision loss right away?" Rosa Garcia asked me. "Now I find out that thou-

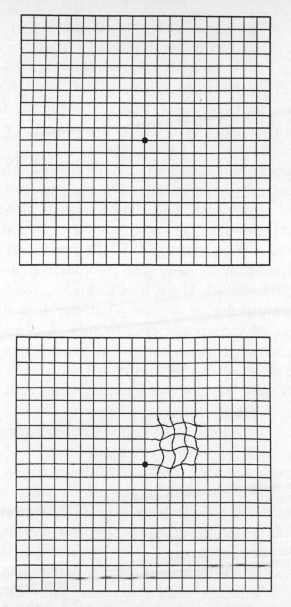

Top: Amsler grid. Bottom: As it may appear to someone with early AMD.

sands of people are checking their vision daily, while I was running around without a clue! Maybe I could have saved my vision, but I wasn't paying careful enough attention." I am here to tell you, as I told Rosa, that it's really not fair to beat on yourself for not noticing changes in your vision.

As chapter 1 explains, your brain is actually hard-wired to ignore changes in your vision by paying attention to your better eye. If blood vessels develop slowly enough in one eye, you are unlikely to notice anything until they leak and cause the distortion or decrease in vision to become very pronounced. Until this happens, your brain will simply decide to see whatever it wants to see out of your other eye. In fact, you may not immediately notice changes in your vision even if you cover each eye and check with an Amsler grid. That's because our visual system is also designed to fill in whatever information seems missing when we look at something. Sometimes your brain will tell you that you see a complete Amsler grid even when your eyes actually perceive wavy lines. This is a wonderful evolutionary adaptation for daily life, but it isn't a great advantage for catching macular degeneration early. However, that is not your fault.

Additionally, because the Amsler grid uses straight lines, it tends to assist your brain in camouflaging any vision loss you might have. Researchers in Israel are developing a better self-test, called the MCPT, that uses dots instead. The MCPT may have an accuracy rate in catching early wet AMD of up to 94 percent, compared with the Amsler grid's 34 percent. Clinical trials are underway on the MCPT, so hopefully we will soon have an even better tool for detecting AMD.

The second unintended side effect is that checking the Amsler grid daily can be very stressful. You are unlikely to get out of bed, sit with one hand over your right eye, peer at the Amsler grid, and discover that your vision has improved. So checking the Amsler grid is like asking whether today is the same as yesterday or worse. It's an exercise in looking for the negative. That's one reason why it's worth asking your doctor whether or not checking the Amsler grid daily is really necessary.

Third, the Amsler grid is too often the only thing people receive when they hear their diagnosis of macular degeneration. This gives many people the impression that the Amsler grid is the only tool available. You stick it on your refrigerator, and then what? While an important test, the Amsler grid has very limited application. It is useful for facilitating early laser treatments that are effective for a certain percentage of people with wet AMD. That's it. It can't provide a prevention plan, nutrition information, research results, visual rehabilitation, emotional coping strategies, or marital counseling for vision loss. It's just a little grid. And people with macular degeneration need a whole lot more than a little grid.

The Traditional Laser Trade-Off

"We had an information open house for people with macular degeneration," a prominent physician admitted to me a few years ago when traditional laser treatment was the only form of laser treatment available. There were one hundred seniors in the audience. Half of them were waving their hands and shouting, "I had Dr. so-and-so, who did four lasers on my eye, and now I'm blind!" "No one explained to me what would happen! I signed a consent form, but no one told me it would get worse!" "They did this laser surgery and I was better off before!" The other half were holding on to their chairs and shouting, "Sit down and let the doctor finish!" I could hardly get a word in edgewise. One of the retinal specialists on our panel went to get a glass of water. He was mobbed. He came running back up to the podium and asked, "Is there a back door in this building?"

Clearly, traditional laser hasn't left a lot of people happy, even those who detected their wet macular degeneration early. Why not? First, laser can't revive severely damaged cells, so it doesn't restore vision. Many people know this before treatment, but it is so hard not to hope anyway, so many people do, and they are disappointed. What laser does is prevent *additional* vision loss caused by existing abnormal blood vessels. Second, laser delays vision loss in 70 percent of the people who receive it. However, 50 percent of these folks experience recurrent bleeding when new abnormal blood vessels grow or old ones reopen, so laser is a temporary, not a permanent, answer.

The biggest drawback of laser, which many people do not fully understand before they undergo treatment, is what I call the blind spot for better vision trade-off. The heat of a traditional laser beam burns a tiny scar in the macula itself, causing a small blind spot, which many people notice. So what does this blind spot look like? It's usually a dark or darkish spot in the area of your vision that was most affected before treatment, but it really varies among individuals. One person may not see it at all, another may simply notice that his or her vision just isn't quite as good as it was before treatment, while a third person may see it and mind it very much. Certainly it's a shock if it's not expected. If you don't receive laser, however, the abnormal blood vessels causing your vision loss may extend all the way underneath the macula. Once they spread, they will cause even larger dark spots in the center of your vision all by themselves. The idea is to cede a little ground to these rogue blood vessels by zapping the tissue where they are and save the surrounding areas. As Neil Bressler, M.D., of Johns Hopkins University describes it, "You are giving someone poor vision to prevent terrible vision." I know this doesn't sound wildly appealing. That's why PDT is such an important new treatment option.

PHOTODYNAMIC THERAPY (PDT) WITH VISUDYNE

With PDT, we no longer have to face the "blind spot for better vision trade-off." As David H. Orth, M.D., professor of ophthalmology at Rush–Presbyterian–St. Luke's Medical Center in Chicago, puts it, "It's the best treatment I've seen in twenty-five years." PDT arrived in 2000, when the Food and Drug Administration (FDA) approved the drug Visudyne, whose chemical name is verteporfin, for use with PDT treatments. Visudyne is a photosensitive dye that allows doctors to use a cool laser light beam, rather than a hot one, thereby eliminating the tissue damage that the heat from traditional laser treatments does to the macula.

PDT begins with an injection of Visudyne, which travels through your bloodstream, illuminating the vessels. Fifteen minutes later, after the Visudyne has accumulated properly, your ophthalmologist treats these vessels with a special laser light. This light activates the Visudyne, causing it to react with the tissue of the abnormal blood vessels to produce free radicals (see chapter 3 for an explanation of free radicals). The free radicals, in turn, close off the unwanted vessels to prevent leakage. Since it's the light of the laser that activates the Visudyne, rather than the heat, a cool laser can be used, which doesn't cause blind spots on the macula.

More good news about PDT arrived in 2001 when clinical trials suggested that up to a third of the people who have the treatment retain a significant amount of their vision for two years after treatment. More studies, like the VIM study (Visudyne In Minimically Classic CNV) are now underway to confirm those results and to see if PDT with Visudyne is equally effective for all forms of wet AMD. In the meantime, Donald C. Fletcher, M.D., of the University of Alabama, a national leader in the field of visual rehabilitation, reported that in his study of sixty-four participants who received PDT with Visudyne up to 42 percent actually wound up with smaller scotomas. A scotoma is a blind spot, an area of the macula that has been damaged and can no longer process visual images. In other words, while these participants couldn't technically see better in the sense that they didn't necessarily test as having clearer vision, they reported that it was easier to do things—they felt as if they could see more, and essentially they could, because their scotomas were smaller.

You might be thinking, with these advantages, why do we bother with traditional laser at all? Why don't we just use PDT with Visudyne and then we could eliminate the blind-spot trade-off? You're right, but the story isn't that straightforward. The answer is a complicated mix of medical studies and Medicare funding, which we explain below.

Will Laser Work for You?

As of 2002, laser treatments have been approved for use only for people with classic pattern wet AMD because medical studies have so far proven them to be effective only for this subtype. If you have the wet type of macular degeneration (also called CNV, meaning choroidal neovascularization, or SRNV, meaning subretinal neovascular membrane), you have either the "classic" or the "occult" pattern or, most likely, a combination of both patterns. Classic CNV is called classic because it was discovered first and is easier to detect. Your ophthalmologist can see it clearly with a fluorescein angiogram. Traditional laser treatments, which use a hot laser beam, were developed to treat classic CNV and early laser research was based only on classic CNV, so we know much more about it than we know about the occult pattern.

Occult pattern CNV is an entirely different bird, and unfortunately, we do not yet have a treatment for it. Occult pattern has more subtle and irregular blood vessel patterns than classic

CNV and is much harder to identify, so it was discovered more recently. Your ophthalmologist can see it best with an indocyanine green angiogram (ICG). Researchers now believe that many people who had traditional laser treatments for classic CNV and then experienced new bleeding in their maculas may also have had occult CNV. The new bleeding may have come largely from the occult pattern blood vessels that remained undetected and untreated.

The question remains: Why don't we discard traditional laser treatments altogether and use PDT with Visudyne for all cases of classic pattern wet AMD? As it turns out, PDT with Visudyne is more expensive than traditional laser, so Medicare and many private insurers will not reimburse for its use with classic pattern wet AMD unless the blood vessels in question are sitting directly under the fovea, at the center of the macula. This would make traditional laser treatments impossible without causing a very prominent blind spot that would make the cure nearly as bad as the disease.

Many times at talks around the country someone has asked the question John Patrick Reynolds put to me last week: "My neighbor had PDT with Visudyne, but my doctor said he wouldn't do it for me. Why not?" As you now know, there are three possible answers. Either Pat has dry AMD or he has classic pattern wet AMD, but the abnormal blood vessels in his macula are not underneath the fovea, so Medicare will cover only traditional laser treatments. Or he has occult pattern AMD and his doctor wasn't comfortable offering him laser before it's approved by the FDA for use with his type of macular degeneration. This last restriction may change in the next year or two as we see more research results on PDT. It may eventually prove to be effective for occult pattern AMD, too.

Experiencing Angiograms and Laser

Your doctor may recommend a fluorescein angiogram or an ICG or both before laser in order to map the abnormal blood vessels in your macula. A fluorescein angiogram makes classic pattern vessels more visible, while an ICG makes occult pattern vessels more visible. You may have your angiogram anywhere from a few minutes to a few days before laser. Both types are very common, essentially painless office procedures, although they may involve dilating drops, a quick injection of numbing medication in the eye to reduce involuntary movement, and an arm injection. Fluorescein and indocyanine green are types of dye that are injected into your arm. They temporarily color the blood vessels in your eye, making both the vessels and their leaks show clearly on photographs of your retina that your doctor or a technician will then take. Most people feel no side effects from angiograms, although occasionally someone becomes mildly nauseated or develops minor hives from the dye. Serious allergic reactions are very rare.

Like angiograms, both traditional laser and PDT can be done in just a few painless minutes in your ophthalmologist's office. You will receive dilating drops again and maybe a quick injection of numbing medication to prevent involuntary eye movement during laser. Then you simply rest your chin and forehead against supports and look straight ahead. You will not feel the laser beam cauterizing the abnormal blood vessels. Your vision may clear somewhat if there was blood in your macula before laser and it drains away. Many people, however, do not notice a difference. If you have PDT, Visudyne is injected approximately fifteen minutes before the laser treatment. Otherwise the procedure is just the same as it is for traditional laser. Some people experience minor side effects from Visudyne such as flashes of light and glare sensitivity, which should subside. Since Visudyne is a light-sensitive drug, you must avoid direct sunlight for several days after treatments. You can usually do this by wearing long sleeves and pants, a hat, and sun block or by staying inside during the day.

The Gas Bubble to the Rescue

Many people with significant bleeding in the macula from wet AMD have preserved some of their vision with a gas bubble treatment. It's a relatively low-tech yet dramatic procedure that effectively clears away leaking blood, thereby saving the surrounding retinal tissue from asphyxiation. Since gas rises, if you inject a tiny gas bubble into the eye and lie facedown, the bubble will rise, pushing on the macula and literally squeezing the blood out. We should probably call it the gas bubble squeegee method. The gas bubble was the ingenious idea of Australian retinal specialist Wilson Heriot, M.D., and was pioneered and refined by Masahito Ohji, M.D., of Osaka University in Japan. In a 1998 interview with the *Ophthalmology Times*, Mark W. Johnson, M.D., of the University of Michigan called it a "delightful procedure" for its simplicity and predicted that it would become the treatment of choice for managing thick blood pools. And it has. Some physicians use the gas bubble in conjunction with an injection of t-PA, a clot dissolver, although it has not been conclusively proven to make a difference. The catch with the gas bubble is that you need to lie facedown for up to ten days in order for the blood to squeeze out. Your retinal specialist may recommend the gas bubble alone or follow-up with laser treatments, depending on the pattern and severity of your AMD.

CATARACT SURGERY AND MACULAR DEGENERATION

Electing to have cataract surgery if you also have macular degeneration has become a tricky decision. Some studies and anecdotal evidence suggest that cataract surgery aggravates wet AMD and may cause it to get worse, although this hasn't been definitively proven. We don't know why this happens, if in fact it is happening. Perhaps the abnormal blood vessels in the macula become aggravated by the inevitable pressure changes in the eye or the intense light exposure that come with cataract surgery. It may also result from a mild postsurgical inflammation. Whatever the reason, it's a concern. With mild cataracts, your doctor can see what's happening with your macula and you can make an informed decision together. With very advanced cataracts, however, the picture gets trickier. You may also have macular degeneration without knowing it, because your doctor can't see through the cataracts to detect the AMD. Once the cataracts are removed, things will appear brighter, but they may not appear clearer. You may also find yourself needing treatment for the macular degeneration. This does not mean that cataract surgery isn't a good thing. It's a wonderful surgery and it saves lots of people lots of sight—but it is important to understand that it can't clear up fuzzy vision from macular degeneration and it may also come with a risk if you already have wet AMD.

WHY MEDICAL PROGRESS SEEMS SO SLOW

If research is progressing so rapidly, why don't we have a cure yet? Why don't we have better treatment options? Why does medical progress seem so slow in spite of all the media reports on new breakthroughs? These are great questions that many people ask. Part of the answer lies in macular degeneration itself. It turns out that AMD is a much more challenging condition to research than other eye conditions, such as glaucoma and cataracts, for several reasons. First, AMD clearly runs in families, but it only affects people later in their lives, which makes it very difficult to collect data on inheritance patterns. We have to wait until the children of the people who have it today are old enough to develop it, too. Then we'll have adequate genealogical data. In the meantime, researchers are working around this limitation by using other techniques to understand the genetic patterns of AMD, like twin or sibling studies (for a discussion of genetics, see chapter 3).

Second, AMD strikes very delicate, intricate tissue way in the back of your eye. It's a whole lot easier to deal with something like a cataract, which clouds the durable, simple lens sitting right inside the front of your eye. We've figured out how to disintegrate that lens, vacuum it right out, and replace it with a new one, but when it comes to the macula, disintegrating and vacuuming just aren't options. We have to develop much more sophisticated methods of handling this complex tissue. Glaucoma is also more straightforward than macular degeneration. We know that high pressure in the eye plays an important role in glaucoma, so we control it in most people by reducing the pressure through careful monitoring, medication, and surgery. We do not yet know what causes macular degeneration. If our theories are correct, the causes are very complex. For these reasons, it will take longer to really find a cure than we wish. But we have every reason to hope that we will figure it out sooner rather than later.

So what about all these new breakthroughs you may hear about in the media? Where are the new treatments they promise? The answer is: in the testing phase. Federal standards mandate careful testing for all new medical treatments before they are approved. This isn't just a matter of avoiding lawsuits or jumping through regulatory hoops. Experimental treatments can leave you with huge medical bills and no improvement, or they can actually cause damage we didn't anticipate. Look at what happened when thousands of women were given Thalidomide in the 1950s to prevent morning sickness before we had adequate testing standards: their babies were born without properly formed limbs. We want to avoid those kinds of surprises in ophthalmology.

So after positive preliminary results, which may be reported in the media, new drugs and surgery treatments are then thoroughly tested in large, long-term, controlled, randomized, double-masked studies before they are federally approved. Whoa! What does all that mean? *Controlled studies* evaluate whether a treatment actually makes a difference by comparing those who receive the treatment with those who don't and controlling all of the other variables that might influence the results. *Randomized* means that participants are assigned randomly, rather than putting all the best cases in one group or another. *Double-masked studies* means that neither the participants nor the researchers know which participants are receiving treatment, so that no one can knowingly influence the outcome. As you might guess, these studies are astronomically expensive and take years to design and complete.

GONE THE WAY OF THE DODO BIRD: THALIDOMIDE, INTERFERON, AND RED WINE

As it turns out, Thalidomide was actually a candidate for treating macular degeneration, along with the drug Interferon and red wine. These are all examples of treatments that have been debunked through careful testing. Since Thalidomide and Interferon inhibit blood vessel growth in the body, researchers thought that they could prevent the abnormal vessels of wet AMD. Allen C. Ho, M.D., led the multicenter, five-year-long AMDATS (Age-Related Macular Degeneration and Thalidomide Study), announcing his conclusive results in 2001. It turns out that Thalidomide has intolerable, though not dangerous, side effects in adults. Interferon was proven to be ineffective a few years earlier by a similar study. Preliminary studies of red wine also found no positive impact, although it was certainly a more palatable treatment than either drug. As research continues, more experimental treatments will also go the way of the dodo bird, but others will remain to help us retain or restore our vision.

PARTICIPATING IN CLINICAL TRIALS AND TRYING EXPERIMENTAL TREATMENTS

Patients and people with macular degeneration from around the country often ask me about volunteering for an experimental treatment study. I know that if I were losing my eyesight today and felt that one of these unapproved approaches might help, I would seriously consider it. But before I took this chance, I would inquire about the reputation of the physician conducting the study and the organization funding it and about the preliminary results. I would never pay money to volunteer. Reputable practitioners and companies do not charge for participation in clinical trials. To find trials that are recruiting, ask your doctor for a referral, visit the NEI's Web site at www.nei.nih.gov, or contact the macular degeneration organizations listed in appendix A. I do encourage everyone who is eligible to participate in reputable studies.

Because approval for new treatments often takes years, some doctors and many patients are tempted to try one now just in case it works. This is particularly true of treatments that have shown positive results in preliminary studies, such as laser for drusen (see "An Answer for Dry AMD: Lasering Drusen"). That may be the right decision for you, but sometimes the risk is not small and neither is the expense, since Medicare won't cover treatments that are not proven. Before you try one, be sure to have a second opinion from a respected retinal specialist and consider the range of possible outcomes.

NEW DISCOVERIES ON THE HORIZON

There is almost a bewildering number of new discoveries, treatments, and studies on the horizon or happening right now. Here you'll find a pre-view of all of the latest work from around the world. For research updates, see the first paragraph of this chapter or appendix E and ask about the studies by name.

New Lasers

AN ANSWER FOR DRY AMD: LASERING DRUSEN

Up until now, we've thought of laser as a treatment only for wet AMD, but it may prove very effective against dry AMD, too. Drusen, as you may recall from chapter 1, are the small yellowish spots in the macula that are the early signs of macular degeneration. Some researchers argue that drusen are like signposts: they tell us that the eye is experiencing macular degeneration. Lasering them may just remove the signposts without slowing down the condition. Other researchers argue that drusen *are* the condition—that they're the abnormal deposits in the macula that actually damage its tissue. If this is true, lasering them may go a long way in preventing vision loss, especially if they are removed early enough. We already know that we can eliminate drusen with laser if we use a low-intensity beam in a special pattern around the macula. R. Joseph Olk, M.D., of the Retina Center in St. Louis found that after lasering of the drusen in sixty-four patients' eyes their macular degeneration didn't progress for at least two years. As Dr. Olk concluded, "It doesn't take a statistician to figure out that this treatment has a dramatic prophylactic benefit."

What it does take, however, is confirmation of these results in randomized, controlled studies, three of which are now underway. The first is the NEI's five-year CAPT (Complications of AMD Prevention Trial) under the direction of Stuart L. Fine, M.D., chairman of the Scheie Eye Institute at the University of Pennsylvania. A second five-year study, the PTAMD (Prophylactic Treatment of AMD), under the direction of Thomas R. Friberg, M.D., of the University of Pittsburgh, is testing whether lasering drusen can actually restore vision, and a third study, directed by Allen C. Ho, M.D., of the Wills Eye Institute in Philadelphia, is combining laser with a drug that inhibits abnormal blood vessel development. We should hear their results by 2004.

As we look back on the research progress of the last few years, we can be very hopeful. The year 2000 was the year of innovative laser treatment for classic pattern wet AMD, 2001 was the year of new vitamin supplement treatment for everyone, and 2003 and 2004 promise to be the years of a new treatment especially for dry AMD.

AN ANSWER FOR OCCULT PATTERN WET AMD: TRANSPUPILLARY THERMOTHERAPY (TTT)

Transpupillary Thermotherapy (TTT) is our best hope so far for treating occult pattern wet macular degeneration with laser. TTT uses a very low-heat beam over a relatively long period of time—a full sixty seconds—much longer than the short zaps of traditional laser treatments. The abnormal occult pattern blood vessels underneath the macula seem to absorb the laser's heat, which then dries them up. Since the heat level is so low, TTT doesn't damage the macula, so there is no blind spot for better vision trade-off with TTT, but it does require a local anesthetic. A large-scale study involving 336 patients in twenty-two cities is now underway to determine whether or not this form of laser is really effective. The study's name is TTT4CNV (Transpupillary Thermotherapy for Choroidal Neovascularization) and results should be released before 2005.

New Surgeries

SUBMACULAR SURGERY: CLEANING UP THE OLD NEIGHBORHOOD

Before PDT, ophthalmologists couldn't treat wet macular degeneration with laser if the abnormal blood vessels grew underneath the fovea, the center of the macula, because the heat from the laser would damage the tissue and cause a prominent blind spot (see "The Traditional Laser Trade-off"). As a result, in the 1990s a number of physicians began developing surgical methods for saving the fovea. With submacular surgery, the idea is to slip underneath the fovea and remove the abnormal blood vessels that are causing the problem—a sort of high-tech neighborhood cleanup. Submacular surgery made its debut a decade ago, but the first patients who tried it experienced too many complications. Since then Michael Lambert, M.D., of Houston and his colleagues have reported promising results using smaller, less invasive incisions. In 2001, the National Eye Institute (NEI) launched the SST (Submacular Surgery Trials), a study in which ophthalmologists from twenty-nine centers across the country are performing the same surgery on 960 patients to see if it is really an effective treatment. We expect the final results in September of 2005.

MACULAR TRANSLOCATION (RETINAL ROTATION): MOVING TO A NEW NEIGHBORHOOD

Macular translocation is an alternative to submacular surgery. The idea is to save the fovea by moving it a few millimeters to a "new neighborhood" so that it can sit atop an area supported by normal tissue. Since this procedure was first described, surgeons have been working hard to make it both safer and more predictable by refining equipment and developing new techniques to address the problems that limited the success of earlier surgeries. For example, rotating the fovea can cause double vision, so some leaders in this field, like Yasuo Tano, M.D., of Japan and Claus and Ute Eckardt, M.D.'s, of Germany have developed combination procedures that pair macular translocation with eye muscle surgery to eliminate this side effect. Several ophthalmologists in the United States are also pioneering variations of macular translocation surgery, including Eugene De Juan, M.D., of the Doheny Retina Institute at the University of Southern California and Hilel Lewis, M.D., chairman of the Cole Eye Institute in Cleveland. A multicenter pilot study is now underway, comparing macular translocation with PDT using Visudyne to see which treatment is best for people with classic pattern wet macular degeneration.

Both submacular surgery and macular translocation are designed to protect healthy foveas, not to restore sight to damaged foveas, so these surgeries must be performed before vision loss from wet AMD becomes too severe. At this late stage, transplants and computerized eyes may be our best future options (see "Transplant Surgery: Getting a New Macula" and "Computerized Eyes: Restoring Lost Vision").

TRANSPLANT SURGERY:
GETTING A NEW MACULA

"What I need is a whole new eye," Buddy Burmester once joked, half-seriously. We don't have the technology to transplant a whole eye yet, but we can transplant sections, like corneas. Researchers are trying to figure out how to transplant retinal cells in order to rejuvenate the macula's support system. The idea is to introduce new cells that will grow healthy replacement parts, just like bone marrow transplants encourage new marrow growth: until now, three types of cells have been used in these experiments: retinal pigment epithelium (RPE) cells, cone cells, and rod cells. More recently researchers have transplanted whole sheets of retina along with its underlying RPE. Researchers know that these cells can be transplanted and that they will survive and grow. What they don't know yet is whether these cells will transmit visual images accurately. One of the most exciting developments in this field comes from researchers at the Rudolf Foundation Clinic in Vienna, Austria. They are working on harvesting a person's own cells from a healthy part of their retina and injecting them under the macula. They have already tried the procedure with fourteen volunteers, who've experienced improved vision.

Researchers in Japan have developed another creative transplant method using iris cells, the cells that give your eye its distinctive shade of brown, blue, or green. They are trying to introduce a gene into iris cells that transforms them into light-sensing cells, which could then be transplanted into a damaged retina to restore vision. At the Schepens Institute in Boston, researchers are working with stem cells, generic human cells that can mature into any type of body cell. They hope to transform these stem cells into replacement rods and cones for the macula. All of these forms of transplant surgery are still in the early stages of development and will not be available for clinical trials for a number of years.

New Nonsurgical Treatments: Edgy Alternatives

MICROCURRENT STIMULATION: BUZZING THE EYEBALL

Microcurrent stimulation, known as Tensmac (Transcutaneous Electrical Nerve Stimulation to the Macula), uses a small battery-operated device called the TENS to deliver low-intensity electricity to the eyelids. Microcurrent stimulation is already an FDA-approved treatment for arthritis and joint pain, but its use for macular degeneration is new. The idea is that the electrical current will increase circulation in the retina and jumpstart the cells in the macula, giving them extra energy to process visual images. Since Tensmac can't rejuvenate severely damaged cells, it has to be done when the macula is relatively healthy and visual acuity is better than 20/100. Tensmac has only a temporary effect, so it must be repeated weekly or monthly indefinitely. There is no real evidence that Tensmac is effective—no comprehensive studies and no consistent anecdotal reports—and treatments can become very expensive. Like rheo-therapy, Tensmac hasn't garnered widespread interest from mainstream medicine, so a formal clinical trial has not been launched as of 2002.

RHEO-THERAPY: CLEANING THE BLOOD

Rheo means flow or stream, so rheo-therapy is a process of improving blood flow in the hopes that this will increase oxygen delivery to the macula. To improve flow, rheo-therapy uses a blood-filtering process called apheresis that removes certain lipoproteins (fats) from the blood. Apheresis is already an FDA-approved treatment for some blood diseases, but its use for macular degeneration is still experimental. Insurance will not cover the costs without conclusive proof of its benefits, and it may cost up to $2,500 per treatment, prompting state health care agencies to worry about fraud. In response, OccuLogix, the distributor of apheresis equipment, undertook a controlled study of 150 patients, which reported such positive results for the first forty-three patients that the FDA approved an expansion of the study. Definitive results should be reported by 2004. If rheo-therapy turns out to be effective, it may officially become a new treatment for macular degeneration.

RADIATION: BLASTING THOSE UNWANTED VESSELS

Radiation combats cancerous tumors by destroying the blood vessels that supply them with oxygen and nutrients. If radiation works against these vessels, could it also work against the rogue blood vessels that develop with wet AMD? In the 1990s, researchers hoped it would, but a decade of studies has said otherwise. In most cases of cancer, you can blast the cancerous area with relatively high doses of radiation without destroying the surrounding area. The eye, however, is very vulnerable. We've had a hard time finding a radiation dose that's strong enough to work but mild enough that it doesn't damage the whole macula. In addition, radiation is very expensive, so it's prohibitively costly to research it. Most U.S. scientists have given up on the prospect of using radiation to combat AMD, but some European scientists are still trying new techniques. We will probably know in the next few years if radiation promises an answer or it will join Thalidomide in the way of the dodo bird.

New Drugs

ANGIOGENICS: THE CULPRITS

There are literally dozens of drugs in testing for macular degeneration. The most promising research focuses on antiangiogenics, which most ophthalmologists believe will become a key part of our treatment of macular degeneration. An angiogenic is a chemical that causes blood vessels to develop, so an "antiangiogenic" is one that stops blood vessels from developing. Our eyes naturally produce angiogenic chemicals when our maculas are deprived of oxygen as a results of poor circulation, clogged support tissue, or perhaps drusen. It is these chemicals that trigger the production of abnormal blood vessels that characterize wet AMD. We can shut down these vessels with laser, but until we figure out how to block the angiogenics, new vessels will grow in their place. This is the reason that laser can't cure wet macular degeneration; it can only delay its progress.

VEGF: THE CHIEF CULPRIT

VEGF (Vascular Endothelial Growth Factor) is the angiogenic our eyes produce that we believe is the main culprit in wet AMD. We know that

VEGF is present during the development of new blood vessels in the retina, and that our retinas produce VEGF when they lack oxygen. Furthermore, injecting VEGF into normal animal eyes produces new blood vessel growth, and antibodies to VEGF, called VEGF blockers, halt the development of those new blood vessels in animals. These findings are very exciting and have led to a number of clinical trials of synthetic and natural VEGF blockers in the United States and abroad. A list of just a few of the antiangiogenics in studies makes a veritable alphabet and numeral soup: AG3340, NX1838, PEDF, PCK412, EYE001, and rhuFabV2. The last two along with anacortave acetate may be the most promising.

PEDF: Using Viruses to Our Advantage

PEDF (Pigment Epithelial Derived Factor) is a natural antiangiogenic produced in the retinal pigment epithelium (RPE), the supportive tissue beneath our retinas. Seniors have less PEDF in their eyes than younger adults, which may explain why they are vulnerable to wet macular degeneration. At the American Academy of Ophthalmology annual meeting in 2001, researchers from Hong Kong reported that mice that receive PEDF injections do not develop abnormal blood vessels in their eyes. Peter Campochiaro, M.D., of the Wilmer Institute, Johns Hopkins University, showed that PEDF prevents blood vessel growth in animal eyes even when Bruch's membrane is ruptured. Bruch's membrane is the protective barrier that keeps blood vessels out of the RPE, so rupturing it usually triggers new blood vessel growth.

The catch with PEDF is that we can't get it into a pill. In order to have more of it, your RPE needs to produce more of it. In order to get the RPE to produce more of it, you need more PEDF genes—so we need to get those genes into your eye. The best way is to give them a ride in a virus that has been emptied of its viral material. So researchers are busy emptying viruses, filling them with PEDF genes, and injecting them into sample retinas. The viruses do what viruses do best: namely, work their way into the cells and drop off the genes. The genes then do their job producing PEDF. A preliminary clinical trial is planned for this procedure to demonstrate that it is safe for use in humans. If that is successful, a Phase II trial will be launched to determine whether PEDF actually works for wet AMD.

PKC412: Taking a Pill Instead

Taking a pill would be easier than injecting a virus, and that's the beauty of PKC412. It's a drug that inhibits blood vessel growth in several ways; blocking VEGF is only one of these. PKC412 has already passed the Phase I safety trials in people with leaky blood vessels from diabetes and is currently in a multicenter, international Phase II trial. This study is exclusively for people with diabetes and does not include anyone with macular degeneration. However, if it works for them it may also be effective in blocking the abnormal vessel development of wet AMD. There should be more news on PKC412 starting in 2003.

EYE001

This drug with the private eye–sounding name works like an antibody to VEGF when it is injected into the eye. It can be used along with photodynamic laser treatments for better results, and may even reduce the chances of requiring laser treatment in the first place. While early studies have shown successful results in fighting abnormal new blood vessel growth with EYE001, there is one problem: it may actually be *too* effective. VEGF turns out to be vital for cardiac health because it prompts our hearts to sprout new blood vessels when they are needed. EYE001 may do such a good job at blocking VEGF that it puts people who take it at risk for heart attacks. Three people in the initial studies of EYE001 suffered attacks, and researchers have not yet discovered whether this was just coincidence or the result of EYE001. As with all of the other drugs under consideration, we will certainly hear more about EYE001 in the near future.

rhuFabV2

Even though it has an unwieldy name, rhu-FabV2 has the most star-power behind it. By the summer of 2002, seventy people had received experimental injections of rhuFabV2, including actor Dabney Coleman, who was so excited about his positive results that he shared his experience in *People* Magazine. Doctors participating in these trials are equally enthusiastic. As Stephen Schwartz, M.D., of UCLA says, "It is a spectacular advance." As with EYE001, rhuFabV2 needs to be taken very soon after vision loss and is only available to participants in clinical trials. If study results continue to be positive, it may gain FDA approval and be available for broader use some time after 2003.

Anacortave Acetate

Anacortave Acetate is a modified steroid that no longer has any actual steroid activity and therefore none of the unwelcome side effects of steroids. It stops the development of abnormal blood vessels in the eye not by blocking VEGF, like the drugs listed above, but by stopping the development of the cells that form the new blood vessels themselves. Results of early clinical trials were so positive that a large multicenter trial is now underway. With so many new drugs offering answers to wet AMD, we are sure to find at least one that will really work. Perhaps it will be anacortave acetate.

ESTROGEN REDUX

We've all heard about estrogen replacement therapy to prevent symptoms of menopause and the onset of osteoporosis, but can estrogen help prevent macular degeneration, too? Mary Haan, Ph.D., of the University of Michigan School of Public Health is conducting a study, called the WHISE (Women's Health Initiative Sight Exam), to discover whether estrogen or a combination of estrogen and progesterone will reduce the incidence of macular degeneration in women over sixty-five. Dr. Haan expects to announce her results in 2005.

NEW VISIONS OF THE FUTURE

David Guyer, M.D., professor and chairman of ophthalmology at New York University and a nationally prominent retinal specialist, is among the many physicians in the United States who believe that improvements in laser technology combined with new drugs are our best bet for effective macular degeneration treatments in the future. Other ophthalmologists and researchers look to new surgeries or nutritional breakthroughs. For those who have already lost vision, though, there must be another answer.

Spinach That Sees

Plants need light to live and we need light to see. Special proteins in plant leaves capture and process light just like our retinal cells also capture and process light. Okay, plants do it for nourishment and we call it photosynthesis. We do it to see and, well, we just call it seeing. But scientists at Oak Ridge National Laboratory have actually identified the protein in spinach that turns light into an electrical signal and are figuring out how to use that protein in our eyes to compensate for damaged retina cells. As Tanya Kuritz, Ph.D., of Oak Ridge explains, this newly identified protein's name is Photosystem One (PS1). In spinach, PS1 acts like an antenna to capture light and as a kind of reaction center to process it. PS1 can be carried into our retinal cells by microscopic transporters called liposomes. There are still many questions to answer about how we can use PS1 in our own eyes, and we eagerly await clinical trials to see if this ingenious and natural remedy can make spinach more powerful than Popeye ever imagined.

Computerized Eyes: Restoring Lost Vision

A computer chip inside your head? Sure enough, researchers are on a fast track to put one there. Twenty-four different centers in the United

States, Europe, and Japan are developing computer chips that can be implanted either in the brain or in the eye. These researchers regularly share ideas at international meetings so that they can all benefit from one another's discoveries. One of those meetings, a semiannual symposium called The Eye and the Chip, happens in my hometown of Detroit. It is sponsored by the Detroit Institute of Ophthalmology under the direction of my colleague and friend Philip C. Hessburg, M.D.

Five of the most prominent researchers in this field are Mark Humayun, M.D., of the Doheny Retina Institute at the University of Southern California; Raymond Iezzi, M.D., of the Kresge Eye Institute at Wayne State University in Detroit; Joseph Rizzo, M.D., of the Massachusetts Eye and Ear Infirmary at Harvard University; Alan Chow, M.D., of Optobionics, Inc.; and Gregg Suaning, Ph.D., of the University of Newcastle, Australia. Dr. Chow and his colleagues have implanted their computer chip in clinical volunteers. As of 2003, the first six recipients have reported no medical or safety problems and two of the six experienced significant improvement in their vision.

Each researcher's model is different. Dr. Chow's model uses several thousand solar cells in a computer chip implanted under the retina. These tiny solar cells send electrical signals to the nerve cells in the retina, which carry them back through the optic nerve to the brain, acting much the same way the cones of the macula do. Since these cells are powered by the light that naturally enters our eyes, there is no need for additional power or electronics, which greatly simplifies the device.

Dr. Iezzi's three-point system uses chemical signals rather than solar power cells. It involves positioning a camera by the eye, implanting a tiny receiver under the skin, and placing a neurotransmitter delivery device on the surface of the retina. The camera sends visual signals to the receiver. The receiver translates these signals into light impulses and sends these to the neurotransmitter delivery device. This device acts like an inkjet printer in the retina, dispensing chemicals with great precision that trigger nerve cells to send these images through the optic nerve to the brain.

Dr. Humayun's model is similar, except that its signal system is electrical rather than chemical. It uses a one-inch camera that sits on an eyeglass frame. The camera sends a wireless signal to a tiny packet of computer chips that is implanted on the surface of the retina. The chips send electrical messages to the nerve cells in the retina, and they carry it back through the optic nerve to the brain. The system is actually similar to the technology used in cochlear implants for hearing.

Dr. Suaning of Australia has the added

challenge in this field of working with a far more limited budget than American researchers. Undaunted, he and his colleague Nigel Lovell, Ph.D., of the University of New South Wales, have proved the adage that necessity is the mother of invention. They have developed an electrode device that can be enclosed in a ceramic capsule similar to those used in pacemakers and in the same position as our natural lens, near the front of the eye. This greatly simplifies the surgery required since the lens is more accessible than the retina.

Is this science fiction? Not at all. These researchers are very enthusiastic. They have great faith that their systems will someday provide sight for those whose maculas are irreparably damaged. They caution us, though, that the first systems on the market will be those that provide only enough sight for people who are blind to see light and distinguish large objects. These early models will help those with conditions such as advanced retinitis pigmentosa. For a computer chip system to be useful for people with macular degeneration, it will have to provide the kind of fine, detailed central vision of the macula. Since demand for these systems is already high, even though they have not yet been fully developed and thoroughly tested, some shady characters on the fringes of the medical world are already advertising hackneyed versions. Beware of anyone who offers a computer eye implant for a price,

especially those sold or surgically implanted outside of the United States or Canada. Respected
researchers never charge for implanting experimental devices (or for any other experimental
treatment for that matter), and all of the computer chip systems are still considered experimental. Someday, though, they'll be mainstream,
and they will offer us something we have never
had before—the opportunity to restore our sight.

High-Tech and Low-Tech:
What We Can Do at Home

No matter how successful high-tech solutions become, our best option will always be prevention.
There is much we can do at home to reduce our
risk of AMD or to minimize its effects once we
develop it. We already know that smoking contributes to AMD. Some researchers and health
practitioners also suspect that macular degeneration may be related to the increase in other pollu-
tants, particularly from pesticides and herbicides,
that we're all exposed to daily in our food and air.
While we have no proof yet that pollution plays a
role, except for cigarette smoke, there is conclusive proof that our diets do. Until this year we all
knew it was good to eat carrots and dark green
leafy vegetables that are rich in lutein, such as
kale and spinach. Now a new landmark nationwide study has shown that vitamin supplements
are effective enough in combating macular degen-

eration to be considered a new treatment, along with PDT and laser. A second groundbreaking study by Johanna Seddon, M.D., and her colleagues at Harvard University has shown that our risk of macular degeneration is significantly higher if we're eating too much of the wrong kinds of oils in our diets and not enough of the right kinds. The wrong oils turn out to be key ingredients in many common packaged grocery products that are familiar staples in our kitchens: canned soups, frozen dinners, chips, breads, microwave popcorn, and even ice cream. How can this be? And how are we supposed to eat without them? We'll answer both these questions and more in the next chapter. In the meantime, though, it's sobering to think that while tens of millions of dollars are spent on finding a cure for AMD, we might just be able to avoid it altogether if we had something different for dinner and took our vitamins.

CHAPTER 3

Genes, Greens, and Oils: The Causes, Prevention, and Natural Treatment of AMD

It sounds funny to recommend
spinach, given the sophistication of
modern medicine, but there's ample,
basic scientific evidence that shows it
is important to the eyes. Physicians
might do patients a service by
prescribing cookbooks.
—Stuart Richter, O.D., Ph.D.

Mother Nature is no less difficult or
more complicated than any other
mother.
—John Breitner, M.D., M.P.H.
Johns Hopkins School of Hygiene and
Public Health

In this chapter, we've put all the known risk re-
ducers together to come up with a five-star pre-

vention program that you can use to help keep your maculas healthy. You'll also find the facts on natural remedies, like wolfberry, and natural practices, like yoga. Perhaps the best news of recent research is this: It's not too late. Even if you already have macular degeneration, you may be able to slow its progress by the choices you make in the grocery store and in daily life. The importance of these choices makes much more sense if we understand the risk factors for AMD and its causes, so we'll begin there.

ARE YOU AT RISK?

Macular degeneration's full name is *age-related* macular degeneration for good reason (there are actually other rarer types of macular degeneration that are not age-related). The number-one risk factor is age. Beyond fifty, the older you get, the more likely you are to develop AMD. Age is followed by smoking, a family history of AMD, blue or light-colored eyes, a diet low in dark green leafy vegetables, and a diet too high in omega-6 fatty acids and too low in omega-3 fatty acids. If you have any of these factors, your risk of developing macular degeneration is greater than if you don't. How much greater? We aren't sure, but greater nonetheless. Besides age, though, these risk factors are not absolutes. You can find smokers with blue eyes, terrible diets, and a family history of AMD who don't have it themselves. You can also find nonsmokers with dark brown eyes, healthy diets, and no family history of AMD who have developed it. But these cases are like the proverbial exceptions that prove the rule. Most people with AMD have one or more risk factors. Why these six risk factors? Why not others? What do these factors have in common? In order to answer these questions, we need to know something about what causes macular degeneration and how free radicals play a role.

THE LEADING RISK FACTORS FOR AMD

1. Age (the older, the higher the risk after the age of fifty)

2. Smoking

3. Family history of AMD

4. Blue or light-colored eyes

5. Diet low in dark green leafy vegetables

6. Diet too high in omega-6 fatty acids and too low in omega-3 fatty acids

WHAT CAUSES AMD?

As chapter 1 explains, macular degeneration is basically a breakdown of the support tissue that maintains the macula. It begins with the accumulation of waste and lipid deposits that clog this support tissue, making it impossible to keep the macula's rods and cone cells clean and supplied with adequate oxygen. Without adequate oxygen, the rods and cones eventually asphyxiate. In wet macular degeneration, abnormal, unstable blood vessels grow through the support tissue, probably in response to this lack of oxygen. Ironically, these vessels are prone to leaks, which flood the rods and cones with blood, asphyxiating them even more quickly. But why does this whole cycle of oxygen deprivation from accumulated waste and lipids begin in the first place? There are two prominent theories that answer this question:

1. Poorly Functioning Blood Vessels

In this scenario, the blood vessels supplying the macula's support tissue do not pick up waste efficiently enough or deliver oxygen consistently enough. As a result, the macula becomes clogged with waste and lacks adequate oxygen. The lack of oxygen kills the support tissue cells and then the rod and cone cells of the macula itself. In the case of wet AMD, new abnormal vessels grow in a kind of misguided effort to supply more oxygen. As we know, these new vessels are weak and prone to leaking, so all they actually wind up doing is wreaking havoc. The question becomes: Why do the original blood vessels become overwhelmed and fail to do their job? The answer may be that the job is too stressful because the waste is too hard to pick up.

2. Abnormal Waste Tips

In this scenario, the real culprit is damaged or abnormal waste. Rod and cone cells have disposable lipid (fatty) tips. When they process light and metabolize oxygen, the tips fall off as waste and new tips grow. Normally these tips are collected from the macula by the RPE—a layer of tissue supporting the macula—and transported on a "conveyor belt" to waiting blood vessels. These vessels flush the waste tips into the bloodstream. But abnormal waste tips lack the handles the RPE uses to identify them and drag them away, so they sit around, taking up space and making it difficult for the RPE to supply fresh oxygen deliveries. The lack of oxygen kills first RPE cells and then the rods and cones. Of course, it may also trigger the growth of abnormal leaky blood vessels. The question in this scenario becomes: What is causing the waste tips to be abnormal?

So which scenario is it? We don't know yet; it may even be a combination of both. But either way, free radicals play a role. Understanding that role explains why age, smoking, blue or light-colored eyes, a family history, and our diets are all risk factors—and it tells us what we can do to reduce our risk.

Free Radicals

Free radicals are oxygen molecules with an electron missing, which makes them unstable. Left to their own devices, free radicals cause trouble by reacting with other molecules in our bodies, preventing them from doing their jobs or actually destabilizing their structures. You may have heard of free radicals before, since they are now believed to play an important role in the development of certain cancers. Free radicals are a normal part of our system. We produce them as byproducts of oxygen metabolism. We metabolize a lot of oxygen in our maculas, so we produce a lot of free radicals there. Mother Nature has provided our bodies with a natural mechanism for handling free radicals. They are usually picked up and carried off by antioxidants, molecules we get from our food that are designed to pair up electrically with free radicals and neutralize them. So we are actually designed to handle a certain amount of naturally occurring free radicals. If this is true, though, how are free radicals contributing to cancer and AMD?

The problem is that pesticides, car exhaust, cigarette smoke, chemical food additives, household cleaners, and excessive unprotected sun exposure, which we wind up eating, breathing, and soaking up in record amounts, also produce free radicals. These free radicals are toxic to our eyes and to the rest of our bodies. They overwhelm our limited supply of antioxidants, especially if we aren't replenishing antioxidants by eating foods that contain them. When this happens, the free radicals are literally free to react with the cones in our macula, producing abnormal waste tips. These waste tips are called abnormal because they are thought not to have the characteristics of natural waste products produced in the eye. They don't look like waste and they don't act like waste, so they can't be grabbed by cleaner cells from the RPE, the tissue that underlies the macula, and carried away. Instead, they accumulate in permanent deposits that gum up the macula. Eventually, they back up the entire system that keeps the macula alive until it can't process any more waste or deliver any more oxygen. It's essentially the equivalent of putting steel ball bearings in a garbage disposal. Nothing happens to the bearings, but the disposal breaks.

Almost every single one of the risk factors we have for macular degeneration can be linked to free radicals. The older we are, the more exposure we've had to environmental toxins, so aging makes sense as a risk factor. The lighter our eyes, the less protective melanin (or pigment) they have to protect us from free radicals produced by the sun, so blue or light-colored eyes make us more vulnerable than brown ones. Dark green leafy vegetables are rich in the antioxidants that our eyes use to counteract free radicals, so a diet low in these vegetables would leave us more vulnerable. Smoking can be described as the activity of overloading our eyes with free radicals, since the chemicals in cigarettes are full of them. And an imbalance of oils in our body can lead to functional weaknesses and lackluster tissue that is generally ill-prepared to handle the free radical onslaught of modern living.

Is Pollution Really a Major Problem?

Yes, I believe it is, but we haven't proved it yet. We are just beginning to understand how pollution affects our health. Cancer, some birth defects, asthma, allergies, and other autoimmune conditions have been linked to industrial chemicals of one kind or another. There is still much research to do on the many unanswered questions, but it looks more and more as if macular degeneration may join this list, making environmental regulations critically important. For our overall health we should demand that legislators protect our air and water and ensure that we have access to accurate information about chemicals used to produce and process our food. Macular degeneration is now appearing in industrialized countries without a known history of the condition, such as Japan and Argentina, which suggests that pollution may play an even larger role than we assume. There is also some evidence that people who live in rural areas with organically grown foods have less risk of AMD. One 1997 study conducted in the isolated mountain village of Salandra, Italy, where residents grew their own food, found that even though 30 percent of the population had blue eyes, their rate of macular degeneration was less than half the U.S. rate.

What About Genetics?

If the environment is so important, why is family history a major risk factor? Isn't genetics the real answer? After all, AMD definitely runs in families. Johanna Seddon, M.D., of Harvard has found that people who have a close relative with macular degeneration are three times more likely to develop it than those who don't. Researchers at the Cole Eye Institute in Cleveland found that if one identical twin has macular degeneration, it is 100 percent certain that the other will develop it, too. In fraternal twins, who are genetically like brothers or sisters, the rate is 50 percent. So if you have a sibling with AMD, you probably have at least a 50 percent chance of developing it yourself. But that doesn't mean that macular degeneration is really a genetic disease in the sense that it's caused by a single bad gene—or even a collection of bad genes. True genetic diseases are relatively rare, but millions of people have AMD—even people with no family history of the condition. So how do we explain the fact that AMD clearly seems to be inheritable?

The answer is that what we're calling age-related macular degeneration is probably a collection of different kinds of AMD with varying characteristics—we just haven't figured out how to distinguish between them. This may explain why people have such different experiences of AMD—different periods of onset, different degrees of vision loss, and different patterns of AMD, either dry, occult pattern wet, classic pattern wet, or a combination. Some kinds of AMD may be more genetically determined than others.

We already know this is true with other forms of macular degeneration in general. For example, we know that Stargardt's disease, which is the juvenile form of age-related macular degeneration, is caused by a mutation of the ABCR (ATP-Binding Cassette Retina) gene. The ABCR gene is a transporter gene. It helps to trigger the removal of waste material, so a defect in it would result in waste material building up in the retina and the RPE, eventually damaging the conveyor belt system that supports the macula. Stargardt's usually develops between the ages of eight and thirty and causes patterns of vision loss to those of very similar, although often less extreme, age-related macular degeneration. In 2001, Richard Alan Lewis, M.D., of Baylor University, who studies families with both Stargardt's and AMD, found an association between AMD and the same mutation in the ABCR gene that causes Stargardt's disease. This is good news since transporter genes often respond to drug treatments that make up for the gene's poor performance and to gene therapy that replaces the defective gene with a healthy one.

But unlike Stargardt's, AMD is not a "monogenic" or one-gene disease. It clearly has multiple causes that interact with one another in complex ways. Even those researchers who focus on finding a gene for AMD, such as Paulus de Jong, M.D., of the Netherlands, suspect that only about a fifth to a quarter of AMD cases result directly from genetics. It seems to take a genetic predisposition plus environmental factors for most of us to actually develop macular degeneration. However, genetics research is progressing at lightning speed (at least as far as research studies go). At the 2001 American Academy of Ophthalmology meeting, Edwin M. Stone, M.D., of the University of Iowa cited six major eye diseases whose genetic causes have been discovered in the last ten years. Age-related macular degeneration may be among the next.

YOUR FIVE-STAR
PREVENTION PROGRAM

You can do five things to reduce your risk of developing macular degeneration or slow its progress if you already have it. First, don't smoke and avoid secondhand smoke in bars, restaurants, and your workplace. Second, wear sunglasses with blue blockers, which block blue light rays. Third, eat a healthy diet with at least five servings per week of dark green leafy vegetables such as spinach and kale. Fourth, eat the right amounts of the right oils. And fifth, take a balanced dose of vitamins and minerals. That's the whole ball game in a nutshell.

Where are you going to find blue blockers? How are you going to add dark greens to your diet without turning into Popeye? What are the right kinds of oils? What vitamins should you take and in what doses? We'll answer all these questions and more as we walk through the program in greater detail. A word of caution, though, before you continue reading: Always check with your doctor before changing your diet or exercise habits. You may have health conditions or medications that will require modifying this program, especially if you smoke, have high blood pressure, heart disease, or diabetes, or are taking Coumadin. Eating excessive amounts of spinach may affect your thyroid, so vary your vegetable intake and remember to eat a balanced diet.

YOUR FIVE-STAR PREVENTION PROGRAM

1. Do not smoke. Avoid secondhand smoke.

2. Wear sunglasses with blue blockers.

3. Eat plenty of dark green leafy vegetables.

4. Choose the right oils and eat them in the right amounts.

5. Take a *balanced* dose of vitamins and minerals.

The First Star: Do Not Smoke

No one should smoke. If you don't smoke, don't start. If you do smoke, stop now. I know that quitting is incredibly difficult and smoking is a great pleasure. But smoking is terrible for your health and for the health of anyone who breathes your smoke. Smoking contributes to cancer, heart disease, emphysema, asthma, and macular degeneration. Smoking adversely affects blood circulation and blood vessel health, making wet macular degeneration more likely. And smoking overloads your eyes with free radicals using up the lutein, zeaxanthin, and vitamins C and E your eyes need to take care of the naturally occurring free radicals produced by oxygen consumption in the macula. Smoking also inhibits vitamins from being processed. I can't say enough bad things about smoking or breathing secondhand smoke, and I can't think of anything good about it, especially not for your eyes. If you must smoke, it is doubly important that you follow the remaining recommendations for reducing your risk of macular degeneration, especially the diet and vitamin recommendations.

The Second Star:
Wear Sunglasses with Blue Blockers

You are probably already aware of the importance of wearing sunglasses with ultraviolet (UV) light protection. This is important since UV rays can contribute to cataracts. But extensive laboratory studies of primates provide persuasive evidence that blue light may be more damaging to the macula than UV light. Blue light waves are visible to us; they're what give the sky or any other object its blue color. Blue light waves are also very short and scatter easily, so a great deal of the glare we experience from sunlight also comes from blue light. Blue blockers are simply a lens tint, usually an amber color, that blocks blue light rays. Unlike other tints, blue blockers don't make the world look darker because they still let in a considerable amount of light while blocking glare. For this reason, blue blockers were very popular a few years ago as sports sunglasses. Many people with macular degeneration find them particularly helpful regardless of their health benefits because they reduce glare indoors and outdoors while keeping the world bright and visible.

WHAT DO WE KNOW ABOUT BLUE LIGHT?

Blue light has been shown to cause a photochemical reaction that produces free radicals in the eyes of primates. Researchers believe that these free radicals may interact in human eyes with the high oxygen and lipid content of the rod and cone tips to produce abnormal chunks of metabolized waste. Melanin, the substance that gives eyes their color, protects the macula by capturing the free radicals produced by light and escorting them out before they cause damage to the macula. People with blue or light-colored eyes or fair skin have much less melanin than people with dark eyes. Light-colored eyes transmit up to one hundred times as much light to the back of the eye as dark eyes do, and they have less melanin to absorb the light's radiant energy. If you have light eyes, you just weren't designed to take in a lot of sun.

Although the laboratory studies on animals

seem nearly unanimous, the real-world studies on people have produced conflicting results. Some studies positively link macular degeneration with any kind of light exposure, while other studies have found a weak correlation. Yet another group of studies has found no correlation at all between macular degeneration and sunlight. One Australian study concluded that the problem may not be how much time you spend in the sun but how sensitive you are to sunlight. It suggested that people who have plenty of melanin and don't tend to burn easily are at less risk for macular degeneration than people who burn easily or are bothered by sun glare, but this study hasn't been replicated. We don't know for sure whether blue light contributes to AMD—but it appears likely. To protect yourself, especially if you have little melanin, wear blue blockers outside.

FINDING BLUE BLOCKERS

The color that blocks blue is yellow, so blue blockers must contain a yellow tint. You can purchase ready-made NOIR sunglasses that block blue and UV light with a variety of tints, including light yellow, dark yellow, orange, amber, and plum. People with macular degeneration usually prefer dark yellow, amber, or plum. NOIR glasses are available as clip-ons or in regular frame styles. Both NOIR and Eschenbach also offer large plastic frames that fit over your regular glasses (see the catalogs listed in appendix C). You can also ask your local optical shop to make you a pair of blue blockers or have your current glasses tinted to block blue light.

The Third Star: Eat Plenty of Dark Green Leafy Vegetables

You may have heard that some fruits and vegetables, such as blueberries, broccoli, and tomatoes, are particularly rich in antioxidants. Many cancer prevention diets recommend broccoli especially. You are unlikely, though, to be eating vegetables that are rich in lutein, an antioxidant important for your macula. These vegetables are less popular and less familiar, particularly outside the South. They are the dark green leafy ones: kale, collard greens, mustard greens, Swiss chard, and spinach. Red peppers and romaine lettuce contain smaller amounts of lutein. Johanna Seddon, M.D., and her colleagues at Harvard University first reported the benefits of these vegetables to our eyes in 1994. They found that people who ate at least five servings per week of dark green leafies had a 43 percent lower risk of macular degeneration than those who ate small amounts or none at all. While this study did not prove that eating vegetables will prevent AMD, its findings were striking enough to get everyone's attention. I wouldn't be surprised if subsequent studies substantiate Seddon's work in the next decade.

I recommend eating exactly what the folks in Seddon's study ate. To do this, you need to have at least five servings of dark green leafy vegetables per week totaling 15,000 micrograms of lutein per serving. A serving is approximately 3.5 ounces or 3 cups of greens uncooked. Since tallying thousands of micrograms and estimating ounces is an impossible task (we've tried it), we've found an easier way. On the following chart, 15,000 micrograms is roughly equal to five points. So if you eat any combination of dark green leafies that adds up to twenty-five points per week, you will get the right amount of nutritional protection and most likely decrease your risk of AMD.

You're probably thinking, Are you kidding? I'll turn green. You might suspect that eating kale isn't going to be a pain-free process. You're not alone. Most Americans aren't used to eating enough vegetables. Our diets have been shaped in part by the now-debunked FDA food pyramid, which emphasizes breads and meats at the expense of vegetables. If you're not a southerner, you may not be used to preparing or eating kale, collard greens, or mustard greens. Not to worry— we've got some fantastic greens ideas in chapter 4. You'll also find our collection of ten favorite greens recipes from friends, family, and the folks at our visual rehabilitation center, as well as ten new simple gourmet greens recipes by Omri Aronow, chef at Rick & Ann's in Berkeley, California.

CHOOSE ANY COMBINATION OF LUTEIN-RICH VEGETABLES THAT ADDS UP TO 25 POINTS PER WEEK*

3 UNCOOKED CUPS OF	GIVES YOU THIS MANY LUTEIN POINTS
Kale or collard greens	7
Spinach, Swiss chard, or cress	4
Parsley (not dried) or mustard greens	3
Red peppers, romaine lettuce, beet greens, or okra	2
Broccoli (2 cups), peas (½ cup), or leaf lettuce	1

* If you eat fewer than 25 points per week, take lutein supplements or a multivitamin with lutein to make up the difference.

We know that even with the best recipes, there may be times when you aren't able to eat enough dark green leafy vegetables to get all of your lutein for the week. Your local grocery store may not have good-quality produce in stock, or you may be too busy to plan and cook, or perhaps your job or life-style requires you to eat out a great deal and your only options are what a restaurant menu offers. If this is the case, try eating at least half of your lutein from fresh or frozen vegetables and getting the rest through supplements. There are a number of multivitamins and minerals on the market today that include lutein.

The Fourth Star:
Choose the Right Oils and
Eat Them in the Right Amounts

Late in 2001, Dr. Seddon and her colleagues at Harvard University reported another startling finding about nutrition and AMD. They found that people whose diets have the right ratio of omega-3 and omega-6 fatty acids have less macular degeneration than those whose diets are skewed. The real bombshell, though, is that most of us are eating skewed diets—*very* skewed diets. We get five times more omega-6 than we should and hardly any omega-3 at all. Since omega-6 and omega-3 compete with each other in our bodies, what little omega-3 we get hasn't got a prayer of protecting our retinas, which is one of its jobs. It turns out that the rods and cones of our macula need a certain amount of omega-3 to function properly. This may be a major reason that so many of us are winding up with accumulated waste in our maculas and AMD.

What are fatty acids anyway? Fatty acids are fat molecules found in saturated fats such as butter and in unsaturated fats such as safflower and olive oil. We all know by now that if we eat large quantities of saturated fats, we'll clog our arteries and we'll wind up as candidates for a heart attack. As a result, many people have turned to vegetable oils for a healthier diet. But large quantities of common vegetable oils, like corn, safflower, and soybean oil, may increase our risk of macular degeneration because they are chock-full of omega-6 fatty acids.

You don't have to eat fried food or use lots of vegetable oil in your cooking to be getting too much omega-6, because these oils are key ingredients in just about every commercial food product on the market, especially low-fat foods such as crackers, sports bars, and microwave popcorn. I recently checked every label in a food mart and found that the only products in the whole store that didn't contain omega-6-rich vegetable oils were the ketchup, mustard, and relish. Everything else that came in a box, bag, can, or package contained omega-6 oils, including the Ben & Jerry's ice cream. To reduce your omega-6 consumption, therefore, you need to avoid packaged foods with vegetable oil listed in the ingredients.

OUR HEROES: OLIVE, CANOLA, FISH, AND FLAXSEED OILS

The right ratio of omega-6 to omega-3 fatty acids is 3:1, which means that we need to consume approximately three times as much omega-6 as omega-3. We already know that vegetable oils such as sunflower, safflower, and soybean are rich in omega-6, but they aren't very healthy choices, especially for cooking, because these oils are polyunsaturated, which means that they don't actually tolerate heat well. Cooking with them degrades their chemical structure, making them possible candidates for producing abnormal waste when they are metabolized in our bodies. So what oils should we use? The answer is monounsaturated oils such as olive and canola oil for their omega-6 fatty acids and fish oil and flaxseed oil for their omega-3 fatty acids.

Omega-6 for Cooking and Baking: Olive-, Canola-, and Oleic-Rich Oils

For cooking, use good-quality olive or canola oil. These oils contain high levels of oleic acid, a monounsaturated oil that tolerates heat and light much better than polyunsaturated vegetable oils do, so cooking won't significantly degrade its nutritional content. If you have a recipe that calls for another oil, check with your health food store. Some of the companies that produce high-quality olive and canola oils also have lines of oleic-rich safflower, sesame, almond, corn, and peanut oils that you can use, especially for baking.

Omega-3 from the Sea: Fish Oils

Cold-water fish, such as sardines, herring, and salmon, are good sources of omega-3 fatty acids. If you buy canned fish, choose it in spring water, not soybean oil, which has enough omega-6 in it to drown out the benefits of the omega-3 in the fish. Some health critics caution that ocean-caught cold-water fish carry high levels of industrial toxins in their fatty tissue. Farm-raised fish are safer, but they often have lower levels of fatty acids, so it's a trade-off. Many people prefer to forgo fish oils altogether in favor of flaxseed oil instead.

Omega-3 from the Land: Flaxseed Oil

Flaxseed oil is one of the world's best sources of omega-3 fatty acids. It has a slightly nutty flavor that makes great salad dressing, especially when it's mixed with your favorite vinegar. Because flaxseed oil is extraordinarily sensitive to light and heat, it comes in a small black opaque bottle with its pressing date and expiration date clearly printed on the label. You can find flaxseed oil in the refrigerated section of a health food or natural grocery store. Two of the best brands are Spectrum and Barlean's, which also market omega-3-rich Norwegian fish oil capsules. Be sure to store these oils in your refrigerator at home or they will spoil, and discard them after they have expired. To increase your omega-3 fatty acid intake, have a serving of fish or fish oil capsules or a tablespoon of flaxseed oil at least three days a week.

AVOID JUNK OILS

No matter what type of oil you buy, avoid the ones in jumbo clear plastic bottles sitting on the grocery store shelves. They're full of oil that's been torched within an inch of its life and has little nutritional content remaining. Oil manufacturers want products that never expire so they can sit in warehouses and stores for weeks or months before they're sold, and then they can sit in your kitchen for as long as you'd like. They never go bad. But we should know by now that food that never goes bad isn't food anymore. It's just an industrial invention masquerading as food. Companies create these nonspoiling oils by blasting them with heat and light, which alters their chemical makeup dramatically. This is especially true of polyunsaturated oils, such as safflower, corn, and soybean oil, which do not tolerate heat or light very well in their natural state. I call them junk oils—they're like liquid junk food in a bottle.

Choose good-quality oils. What is a good-quality oil and how do you know it when you see it? A good-quality oil is one that hasn't been processed out of its natural state, so that it's still rich in nutrients and not chemically altered. Knowing it when you see it can be tricky. Oils that say "cold-processed" or "expeller-pressed"—processing methods that avoid heat—are better bets, as are oils with some natural color or with expiration dates, but it's sometimes hard to tell what's been heavily processed and what hasn't, regardless of what the label claims. Your best bet is to shop for oils at a health food store or natural grocery that carries high-quality brands with good reputations in the natural health community.

AVOID PARTIALLY HYDROGENATED OILS

An even more insidious problem than heavily processed oil is partially hydrogenated oil. These are the oils used in most packaged foods. Not only are they rich in omega-6 fatty acids, but they've been chemically altered into little Frankenstein monsters. Partially hydrogenated vegetable oil is created by adding hydrogen to a vegetable oil molecule. This chemical alteration allows the vegetable oil to remain solid at room temperature, like margarine and shortening, which are the Adam and Eve of hydrogenated products. These altered oils can then be substituted for solid saturated fats, such as butter, which is why they're used in lots of "low-fat" foods. Hydrogenation was a great invention, it seemed. It allowed the packaged food industry to boom, and it seemed totally healthy and safe. But it's not.

The problem is that partially hydrogenated oil is not a substance that occurs in nature—it's totally artificial. When partially hydrogenated oil is digested and metabolized in your body, it produces waste products like all other nutrients do. But these waste products are deformed, so the body doesn't know what to do with them. They don't have the normal chemical signs on them that say, "I'm a waste product; throw me out!" And they don't have the normal handles that the cleanup cells use to haul them away. (You can almost hear the cell cleanup crew at morning coffee break: "Hey, Bob, I saw some of those strange blobs out there again, but I don't have any orders to pick them up, so I left them there.") So these weird waste products sit there, accumulating like hair in the bathtub drain or steel ball bearings in the garbage disposal, clogging up the system. After a while, if there are enough of them, they damage the tissue around them by making it impossible for that tissue to clear away its own waste or to get enough oxygen. Sounds familiar, doesn't it? And there's no way to get rid of these blobs. The answer is to avoid eating them in the first place.

CHOOSING THE RIGHT OILS

1. Shop for oils at your health food or natural grocery store. Choose expeller-pressed or cold-pressed brands.

2. Take a tablespoon of flaxseed oil or a serving of fish or fish oil capsules at least three times a week.

3. Use olive oil or canola oil for cooking.

4. Use oleic-rich, monounsaturated vegetable oils for baking.

5. Avoid packaged foods made with vegetable oil, especially partially hydrogenated vegetable oil.

6. Don't use margarine or vegetable shortening.

The Fifth Star:
Take a *Balanced* Dose of
Vitamins and Minerals

In 2001, the NEI announced the results of its groundbreaking ten-year study of vitamins and macular degeneration, the AREDS (Age-Related Eye Disease Study). More than 3,700 people participated from around the country under the direction of the NEI's Division of Epidemiology and Clinical Research. This study proved beyond a doubt that vitamins work if you already have macular degeneration. In fact, they work so well that they can now be considered a treatment, along with laser treatment. The AREDS showed that people with moderate or advanced AMD who took beta-carotene, vitamin C, vitamin E, zinc, and copper, in the doses listed in the box, had a 25 percent lower risk of their macular degeneration progressing than those who took none of these. The AREDS was launched in 1992, before lutein and zeaxanthin were thought to be important nutrients for our eyes, so they were not included in the study, nor was selenium. It is possible that with these additional supplements, the success reported by the AREDS would have been even greater.

If you already have full-blown macular degeneration it's essential to start taking a good-quality multivitamin and mineral supplement. If you are at high risk for macular degeneration or if you have early signs of it, supplements may help prevent its development or retard its progression, although this hasn't yet been definitively proven. Nevertheless, why wait? Now's a good time to choose a multivitamin and take it regularly.

RECOMMENDED VITAMINS AND MINERALS AND THEIR DOSES

Beta-carotene	25,000 IU (not if you smoke)
Vitamin C	500 mg
Vitamin E	400 IU
Zinc	60–80 mg
Copper	2 mg
Lutein	10 mg (take at different time from beta-carotene)
Selenium	200–250 mcg

CHOOSE GOOD-QUALITY SUPPLEMENTS

Although taking any vitamin or mineral supplement is likely to be better than taking none at all, there are good reasons for choosing natural vitamins that are cold processed and that use vegetable coatings rather than food varnish coatings. Cold processed means that the nutrients in the vitamins have not been subjected to high levels of heat during manufacturing, which minimizes their effectiveness. Vegetable coatings are easier on your digestive system and do not contain as many artificial ingredients as varnish coatings. However, most vitamin labels don't give you information on their coatings or processing methods. In fact, since the FDA does not regulate vitamins or minerals, none of the claims on their labels are actually monitored or verified. Different brands also use different quality ingredients as well as different coatings and production processes, which is one reason why prices vary so greatly (although the most expensive is not necessarily the best).

So what should you do? Start by narrowing your choice to brands sold at health food specialty stores or natural grocery stores or by asking your doctor or naturopath. Many physicians are not familiar with various brands or do not realize how much they vary in quality, but your doctor may know. In fact, some of the best brands are now sold through physician's offices. You can also consult an independent evaluator, such as Consumer Reports (www.consumerreports.org) or ConsumerLab.com.

In addition to the nutrients and doses listed in the box, consider choosing supplements that include any or all of the following: zeaxanthin, grape seed extract, gingko biloba, bilberry, taurine, N-acetyl cysteine, and glutathione. On many vitamin packages, vitamin A is included in beta-carotene, since some beta-carotene becomes vitamin A in the body. Lutein may also be listed as part of the beta-carotene complex.

AVOID EXCESSIVE DOSES

Vitamins and minerals do not work alone in our bodies, and neither can any other kind of nutrient. They always need the whole team of players found in a wide variety of fruits and vegetables. Just taking vitamins C and E or a lutein pill or adding spinach to a diet of coffee, steak, chips, and ice cream is like asking Phil Rizzuto to field hits from an entire lineup of free radicals and win the game all by himself. He may be a fabulous player, but he will lose every time. You need the whole complement of nutrients that your body was designed to use, and you need them all in balanced amounts.

For this reason, no one should take excessive doses of any vitamin or mineral. As a rule of thumb, supplements that provide anywhere from the RDA (Recommended Daily Allowance) to two or three times the RDA are best. You may take more of vitamin C or E, since their RDAs are often considered very low and moderately higher amounts of these vitamins are not considered hazardous. The RDA for each vitamin is listed on the bottle along with the percentage of the RDA that each dose provides. If you smoke, avoid high doses of beta-carotene. Drink plenty of water, too. Your body needs water to survive; it's our very first "nutrient." Drinking six to eight glasses of water a day will go a long way in helping your body utilize the vitamins that you've taken to repair its tissue.

THE BEST FOUNDATION: A FRESH, VARIED DIET

We look good and we live a long time, but we don't really eat well. Just taking vitamins with a diet of steak, potatoes, and coffee or just taking vitamins with a diet of salad, croutons, and diet Coke isn't a recipe for good health. We habitually eat pretty narrow diets—the same few vegetables or the same frozen dinners year in and year out. We aren't getting the wide range of nutrients we need in our foods to keep our bodies essentially robust. Indigestion, heartburn, allergies, constipation, irritable bowel syndrome, hemorrhoids, high blood pressure, heart disease, some forms of diabetes, some cancers, and very likely macular degeneration are all completely or partially diet-related conditions. It probably isn't an accident that these are our primary health problems today and we experience them at near epidemic levels.

In 1990, the Second National Health and Nutrition Examination Survey revealed that fewer than 10 percent of Americans consumed five servings of fruits and vegetables a day, which is now the recommended amount. Fifty percent consumed no garden vegetable, 70 percent no fruit or vegetable rich in vitamin C, and 80 percent consumed no fruit or vegetable rich in antioxidants that neutralize the free radicals implicated in many cancers and macular degeneration. Few of us are getting the RDA of key vitamins and nutrients in our diets—and the RDA is not the optimal amount but the minimum amount necessary to avoid diseases or conditions caused by deficient diets. In other words, most of us walk around chronically malnourished, despite appearances. Vitamins are effective and often necessary supplements, but the are no substitute for a good foundation: a fresh, varied diet rich in vegetables and fruits.

How We Wind Up Eating Poorly

While we don't set out trying to avoid nutritious foods, it's incredibly easy to do so. First, we often live fast-paced lives that allow a limited time to choose food and prepare it. With less time, it's harder to be creative; we tend to rely on the same old familiar meals. We also tend to rely on snack foods or packaged food, which do not provide adequate nutrition or variety. Second, we don't really understand the importance of fresh fruits and vegetables. We usually think of fruit as something we add to pies or cereal. We think of vegetables as side dishes to meat, poultry, or fish. But fruits and vegetables should be our main dishes, while meat, poultry, fish, and starches should be our side dishes. This takes some rethinking of what breakfast, lunch, and dinner should look like. Third, we don't realize how varied in fruits and vegetables our diets need to be. We often rely on a handful of favorite vegetables that we eat frequently, avoiding all the others or eating them rarely. When I sat down and assessed my own diet a few years ago, I discovered that I regularly ate peas, broccoli, and spinach salads, but that was virtually it for vegetables or fruit. My diet would have been okay if every vegetable contained every nutrient we need. Eating would then be a matter of quantity rather than variety, but this isn't the case.

Ironically, our vitamin-poor diets may be the result of the great availability of food in the United States. With refrigeration, worldwide shipping, hothouses, and industrialized farms, we can eat almost anything in any season. If spinach and red peppers were only available two months out of the year, we would be excited by their arrival. They might even be our only vegetable options during those two months, and we would eat them in greater quantities. But when vegetables and fruits are available year round, they lose their seasonal appeal and we tend to overlook them, choosing only our favorites month after month.

Medicine has contributed to our poor eating patterns by focusing on pharmaceutical and technological solutions to our health problems while overlooking nutrition. We've been running our cars on poor-grade gasoline and oil and then paying the mechanics to fix the problem. And the mechanics haven't been telling us to take care of our cars, at least not as much as they should. I count myself among those mechanics. I only started to talk seriously to my patients about nutrition a few years ago. But nutrition is clearly one of the most important things I can talk about, even when it comes to macular degeneration.

Eating Well

Outlining an optimal diet would take more room than we have in this book, but I encourage you to use other sources to help you create your own. There are many nutrition plans on the market. I recommend using one that emphasizes eating plenty of fruits and vegetables and the right oils and minimizes chemicals or additives in your diet. My favorite plan is Andrew Weil, M.D.'s popular *Eight Weeks to Optimal Healing Power*, which provides easy-to-follow guidelines. His book is available in print and audiotape.

At the Very Least, Get the Big Seven

If you decide not to follow a nutrition program or plan, you should at least make sure you are regularly eating foods that give you a natural source of the big seven: beta-carotene, lutein, vitamins C and E, selenium, zinc, and copper. To help you add these foods to your diet, here's a partial list of sources for these nutrients:

NUTRIENT	SOURCES
Beta-carotene	red peppers, carrots, avocados, asparagus, squash, sweet potatoes, nectarines, apricots, cantaloupe, mango, papaya, watermelon, kiwi, and dark green leafy vegetables
lutein	kale, collard greens, mustard greens, spinach, parsley, Swiss chard, and romaine lettuce
vitamin C	red and green peppers, broccoli, Brussels sprouts, turnips, cabbage, citrus fruits, cantaloupe, kiwi, and dark green leafy vegetables

NUTRIENT	SOURCES
vitamin E	seeds, nuts, and whole grains
selenium	wheat germ, oats and bran, fish, egg yolks, chicken, garlic, and red Swiss chard
zinc	oysters and fish, pumpkin seeds, ginger root, pecans, and Brazil nuts
copper	Brazil nuts, almonds, hazelnuts, walnuts, pecans

HEALING FRUITS

Wolfberry (Gou Qi Zi): China's Berry for Your Eyes

While you may be familiar with lutein, you probably haven't heard much about zeaxanthin and have heard nothing at all about wolfberry (lyceum barbarum). Lutein is a key antioxidant for your eyes. It occurs in high concentration in the rod cells of your retina, which are largely responsible for your peripheral vision. But the cone cells of your macula, which allow for detailed central vision, have high concentrations of zeaxanthin. Lutein and zeaxanthin are sister pigments. They protect your retina by neutralizing the free radicals from sunlight that may damage eye tissue. There are very few foods rich in zeaxanthin. Wolfberry is one of them.

Wolfberry is a sweet mild fruit that the Chinese have used to ensure healthy eyes for nearly two thousand years. Mark O. M. Tso, M.D., D.Sc., of the Wilmer Institute of Johns Hopkins University calls it the "Chinese Chicken Soup for the Eye." Sure enough, Dr. Tso discovered that rats that eat these berries (which they love) do not suffer damage to their maculas when they are exposed to strong light, a strong sign of the preservative powers of zeaxanthin. Dr. Tso has launched a clinical study to discover whether wolfberry will also protect the maculas of humans, in hopes of developing a much-needed treatment for dry macular degeneration. Wolfberry may also have beneficial effects on the liver and immune system.

Dried wolfberries are small and sweet like raisins. You can stew them with meats (add wolfberries ten minutes before the meat is done) or steam them with chicken or fish. You can also add them to nut or dried fruit mixes, sprinkle them on cereal, add them to bread, muffin, or pudding recipes, boil them to make tea, or enjoy a few tablespoons as a mid-afternoon treat. To find them, ask a Chinese grocery or certified Chinese medicine practitioner for Gou Qi Zi or contact a Chinese foods and herbs import company such as Rich Nature (www.richnature.com, 425-774-2266).

Bilberry:
The RAF Pilots' Secret Weapon

During World War II a group of Royal Air Force (RAF) pilots demonstrated almost supernatural night vision by downing shadowy Luftwaffe fighters during pitch-black raids with devastating accuracy. Legend has it that the secret to their success was bilberry jam. Bilberry, a British cousin of the huckleberry, is said to enhance night vision and, because of its deep pigment and bioflavonoid qualities, may help repair eye conditions associated with cell damage, such as cataracts and macular degeneration. But limited studies conducted in the last ten years have not confirmed these claims. And it turns out that, rather than berries, the pilots' secret may actually have been radar, which the British developed in the middle of the war. Not wanting the Axis powers to discover its use, the RAF put out the word that the pilots' diet was enhancing their eyesight. Does this mean that bilberry is a dud? Not necessarily. It may have strong medicinal powers, but we just don't have the proof. If you'd like to try bilberries, look for bilberry jam at your local specialty food store or natural grocery store and spread it on your toast in the morning.

Noni Juice:
The Polynesian Tonic

For thousands of years, the people of the Polyne-
sian islands have used the juice of the *noni* fruit
as a skin salve, antioxidant, and immune system
enhancer. While there is no scientific proof of *noni*
juice's healing powers, you can find it in your local
health food store and some physicians suggest it
for their patients. *Noni* juice has never been stud-
ied in relationship to AMD, although I have seen
one anecdotal account of its beneficial effects by
a woman with Stargardt's, the juvenile form of
macular degeneration. If you would like to try
noni juice, you can find it at your local natural
grocery or health food store. Of all the healing
fruits associated with your eyes, though, I believe
wolfberry will turn out to be the most important.

HEALING PRACTICES

Some folks put microstimulation and rheo-therapy
in this category, but we talk about them in chapter 2 instead. Anytime you're applying electrodes
to your eyes or running your blood through a
machine, I don't think it can really be called
a natural treatment. But there are many other
practices people are using to heal their bodies
that are holistic: meditation, yoga, tai chi,
acupuncture and acupressure, massage, saunas

and steam baths, and exercise. Are they effective for macular degeneration? Honestly, we don't know. There hasn't been a formal study on any of these practices as a treatment for AMD. However, there have been plenty of studies confirming their beneficial effects for the body as a whole; this is particularly true of meditation and yoga. There is no reason to believe that a healthy body wouldn't contribute to healthy eyes and to a healthy spirit as well.

Yoga and Meditation

I love yoga. Yoga is essentially a meditation practice that centers your mind through specific body movements. Some forms of yoga, such as power and Ashtanga yoga, are extremely athletic and not relaxing at all, unless you are made of rubber, but others are very healing for both the mind and the body. Iyengar yoga, for example, is particularly good if you are stiff or have previous injuries. Many yoga teachers will combine movements from different schools of yoga to offer the best approach for their students. If you are in any doubt, call and ask to speak to the instructor ahead of time. He or she should be able to recommend the best class for you and tell you what to expect and what to wear. If you have low vision, tell your instructor so that he or she can give clear verbal directions. The best instructors will listen carefully to your concerns and allow for voluntary rest time during class so that you can follow the movements at your own pace.

Meditation alone has many of the same benefits as yoga: it can lower your blood pressure, reduce your stress, enhance your sleep, and support your body's natural healing process. Just as there are many forms of yoga, there are also many forms of meditation. One of the most popular is "mindfulness" meditation, which focuses on simply becoming completely aware of the thoughts in your mind, without any judgment. It's very hard to learn on your own. For this reason, it's often best to learn meditation in a class, even though it's essentially a solitary practice. Many people who have meditated for years regularly do so in advanced classes or meditation workshops for company and encouragement. Meditation and prayer have much in common. If you are religious, consider committing to a regular practice of prayer in your life. This, too, can be a powerful healer. One note of caution: If you are experiencing depression, avoid meditation. As someone once put it, when you're depressed, your mind is like a bad neighborhood—you don't want to go there alone. You need to move your body instead: aerobic exercise and yoga are good antidotes for depression (see chapter 6).

The Bates Method

William H. Bates first publicized his method of treating poor eyesight with eye muscle exercises in 1920, and it's been very controversial ever since. It's also inspired many similar approaches, such as Eye-Robotics, Visionetics, and the See Clearly Method, although none so famous. The Bates method includes various activities like shifting one's gaze between focal points, swinging the neck and head, juggling balls, and allowing sunshine to warm the whites of one's eye through closed lids, which are designed to stimulate circulation in the eyes or to retrain the eye muscles. Despite its perennial popularity, though, there is no medically accepted evidence that the Bates method or any similar program actually works.

I have read a handful of anecdotal accounts by people with macular degeneration who say that the Bates method has helped them see better or read a line lower on the eye chart. What happens to a few folks who try the Bates method or another version may be similar to what happens to everyone in visual rehabilitation: they learn to use the vision they have more effectively. As for the theory that better circulation to the retina would help with AMD, that's probably true, but it's unclear that the Bates method would guarantee better circulation. Since our eye muscles are not connected to our maculas—they do not share the same blood vessels—moving these muscles alone won't help. It takes moving the head, neck, shoulders, torso, and perhaps the whole body, as we do when we exercise or take yoga, to really get our blood moving.

CHAPTER 4

New Gourmet Greens: Recipes for Your Eyes

You probably already eat spinach, red peppers, and romaine lettuce. But unless you're a southerner, the dark green leafy vegetables that are rich in antioxidants for your maculas aren't likely to be familiar to you. Many people admit they wouldn't recognize kale if it were walking down the street, much less know what to do with it in the kitchen. My father, who has macular degeneration, set out to eat more kale but complained that kale stalks were awfully stringy and tough when you ate them raw.

"Kale stalks?" I asked.

"Yes," he replied. "Kale doesn't seem to have much in the way of leaves, so I eat the stalks."

I imagined a typical kale bunch with long, thick bluish-green leaves.

"Look!" my father exclaimed, taking a big bag of fresh parsley out of the refrigerator.

"Well," I said, "parsley's good for you, too."

Even if you can pick kale out of a crowd, you may still have a creeping suspicion that it would taste rather unsavory. Despite Popeye, dark green leafy vegetables have never had the same appeal as a fine steak. The good news, though, is that dark greens are actually exceptionally easy to embrace. Unlike many other vegetables, most dark greens have a mild flavor that blends well into sandwiches, salads, soups, and pastas. You can add them to your own cooking without changing the flavors you love. And dark greens can be delicious on their own, too.

New Greens Recipes

We're very excited to share a new collection of recipes for dark green leafies in this chapter. Here you'll find ten of our favorites from friends, including Monica and Ken's popular Many Greens Soup from the first edition. We also have a brand-new collection of ten gourmet greens designed especially for you by Omri Aronow, chef at Rick & Ann's in Berkeley, California. Please share them with your family and friends, swap them for new recipes, and spread a love of greens!

Low Vision and Gourmet Greens

If you have low vision, the easiest way to add dark greens to your diet is to use the following suggestions for adding them to familiar recipes for main dishes, soups, sandwiches, and salads. You can also cook them separately using the "Favorites from Friends" recipes. Most of the gourmet recipes in this chapter are also very easy. If you or your friend or family member has low vision, take this chapter to a photocopy shop and have it enlarged to an easily readable print size. Collect these recipes with other large-print recipes in a handy binder. Chapter 14, "Saving Sight at Home and in Your Community," has helpful cooking and magnifier tips for the kitchen.

Using Dark Greens in Your Cooking

Dark greens are generally mild and blend well with other foods. Use them in place of fresh lettuce to add zip to salads and sandwiches. You can interchange any of the greens in this chapter's recipes. If you dislike chard or can't find kale at the supermarket, you can use spinach or mustard greens instead, and vice versa. Fresh, healthy greens should not have a strong odor. If you notice a strong odor, your greens may not be fresh or you may be cooking them for too long. If you like your greens milder, you can blanch them for several seconds in boiling water or, for kale, cook briefly in salted water or broth for one minute before using. Be careful not to overcook, since overcooked greens may not be very tasty.

EYE-HEALTHY DARK GREENS AND VEGETABLES

kale	beet greens
Swiss chard	spinach
cress leaf	parsley
okra	red peppers
collard greens	romaine lettuce
mustard greens	

Adding Dark Greens to Your Menu

- Toss mustard greens and spinach into your regular salads.

- Choose Caesar or spinach salads over iceberg lettuce salads.

- Substitute mustard greens and spinach for lettuce in almost any sandwich.

- Add red-pepper flakes to spaghetti sauce, sandwiches, and salads.

- Add Swiss chard stems to your favorite soups or chowders.

- Add a handful of chopped kale or mustard greens to scrambled eggs or an omelet.

- Add a cup or two of dark greens to your favorite casserole before baking.

Buying and Storing Dark Greens

When choosing your greens, select bunches that are firm. Leathery, wilted, or yellow leaf edges and a strong smell are sure signs that the bunch has been sitting for too long. Fresh greens will store well in the refrigerator for a few days, especially if you wash them, dry them thoroughly, and store them in an airtight Tupperware container. Greens grow in loose, open bunches, so they collect a lot of dirt. Be sure to rinse them well on both sides or soak them in a sink-full of cold water. You can dry them in an inexpensive plastic salad spinner or place them in a colander to drain and then press them with a paper towel.

Measuring and Chopping Greens

Bunches of greens come in varying sizes. Some recipes simply call for a "bunch." Choose whatever size you feel is best or whatever size is available. For recipes that call for chopped or shredded greens, consider using scissors and cutting them rather than using a knife.

FAVORITES FROM FRIENDS

Colleen's Strawberry Spinach Salad

6 cups spinach leaves, chopped
1 cup sliced strawberries
½ cup blueberries
1 (11-ounce) can mandarin oranges, drained
½ cup poppy seed salad dressing
1 tablespoon lemon juice
1 teaspoon sugar (optional)
½ cup toasted walnuts

Combine the spinach leaves, strawberries, blueberries, and oranges in a salad bowl and toss to mix. Mix the poppy seed dressing, lemon juice, and sugar in a bowl or place in a shaker and shake to mix well. Drizzle the dressing over the salad and toss to coat. Sprinkle with walnuts.

Serves 4.

Katie's Easy Kale

1 pound mustard greens or kale
oregano, garlic, onion, lemon or lime juice,
    wine vinegar, and/or nutmeg to taste

Remove stems of mustard greens or kale. Wash thoroughly and boil in 1 inch of water in covered pot for 5 to 10 minutes or microwave. Add any one of several of the following: oregano, garlic, onion, lemon or lime juice, wine vinegar, or nutmeg to taste. Our favorite is nutmeg.

Serves 4–6.

Clare's Easy Chard

1 bunch Swiss chard
1 tablespoon extra-virgin olive oil or
    canola oil
1 tablespoon water
basil, nutmeg, or oregano to taste

Chop chard leaves and slice stems crosswise. Put oil in pan and heat 1 minute. Add 1 tablespoon water and the greens. Cover and cook 2 minutes. Add your choice of basil, nutmeg, or oregano to taste.
    Serves 4–6.

Molly's Spinach-Stuffed Mushrooms

8–12 large mushrooms
1 bouillon cube
½ cup water
1 package frozen spinach, drained
½ teaspoon basil
¼ teaspoon dill weed
¼ teaspoon garlic powder
1 tablespoon grated Parmesan cheese
½ teaspoon salt
pepper

Separate the mushroom caps from the stems. Chop the stems and place in a saucepan with bouillon cube and water. Simmer for 5 minutes. Strain out the stems; set them aside. Simmer the caps in the bouillon liquid for 2 minutes. Strain out the caps and pour bouillon liquid into an 8-by-8-inch pan and set aside. In a separate bowl, combine spinach, mushroom stems, basil, dill, garlic powder, and salt, and mix well. Divide this mixture into the mushroom caps and sprinkle with cheese and pepper. Bake stuffed caps in pan at 350 degrees for 20 minutes.

Serves 4–6.

Suzy's Stir-Fried Greens

    1 bunch of kale, spinach, or collard or turnip
       greens
    1 teaspoon corn starch
    ½ teaspoon ground ginger
    ⅛ teaspoon garlic powder
    1 teaspoon soy sauce
    ⅓ cup water

Wash, drain, and chop greens. Place them in a frying pan. Mix the other ingredients together in a bowl. Pour the mix over the greens and stir-fry.

Serves 4.

Sally's Stir-Fried Greens

    1 bunch of kale, spinach, or collard or turnip
       greens
    2 tablespoons olive oil
    bread crumbs
    salt and pepper to taste
    lemon or lime wedges

Wash, drain, and chop greens. Pour olive oil in frying pan and add bread crumbs, salt, and pepper. Add greens and stir-fry. Serve with lemon or lime wedges.

Serves 4.

Lynne's Spinach Squares

2 packages frozen chopped spinach
¼ cup butter
3 eggs
1 cup milk
1 teaspoon salt
1 teaspoon baking powder
1 pound grated cheese (your favorite)

Thaw and drain the spinach and press out extra water with a paper towel. Melt the butter in a 9-by-13-inch pan. Beat the eggs and add the milk, salt, and baking powder and mix. Add the spinach and grated cheese and mix. Pour the spinach mix into the buttered pan. Bake at 350 degrees for 35 minutes. Cut into squares and serve. Can be frozen and reheated on a cookie sheet at 325 degrees for 12 minutes.

Makes 12 squares.

Anne's Spinach with Watercress

1 bunch spinach
3 bunches watercress
3–4 tablespoons butter
⅓ cup cream

dash nutmeg
salt and pepper to taste

Rinse spinach and watercress thoroughly, drain well, and remove stems. Place spinach, watercress, butter, and cream in large saucepan or soup pot. Add nutmeg, salt, and pepper. Cook over medium heat, stirring constantly, until greens are fully wilted (about 7 to 9 minutes). Serve immediately. Serves 4–6.

Carol's Great Greens 'n' Garlic

1 pound kale or collard greens
¼ cup olive oil
¼ cup garlic, peeled and thinly sliced
½ teaspoon red-pepper flakes
salt to taste and freshly ground black pepper
lemon wedges

Wash greens, cut stems into 1-inch pieces, and chop leaves coarsely. Leave greens wet. In large saucepan put olive oil, garlic, pepper flakes, salt, and pepper. Cook over medium heat for 1 minute. Add greens to saucepan and cover. Cook over medium-high heat for 5 minutes. Greens should still be a little firm. Uncover and continue cooking and stirring over medium heat until liquid is almost gone and greens are tender. Don't overcook. Serve with lemon wedges. Goes very well with fish.
Serves 4–6.

Monica and Ken's Many Greens Soup

1 tablespoon olive oil
1 large yellow onion, finely chopped
1½ teaspoons salt
freshly ground black pepper
4 garlic cloves, minced or pressed
1 large potato, peeled and diced
2 large carrots, peeled and diced
3½ cups chicken stock or 2½ cups chicken
    stock and 1 cup milk
¼ cup white wine
1 bunch kale, stems removed and leaves
    shredded
1 bunch chard, stems removed and leaves
    shredded
1 bunch spinach, stems removed and leaves
    shredded
grated Parmesan cheese

Heat the olive oil in a medium soup pot. Add the onion, ½ teaspoon salt, and a few grinds of pepper to taste. Sauté over medium heat until the onion is soft, about 5 to 7 minutes. Add the garlic, potato, and carrots. Sauté until the vegetables are heated through, about 5 minutes. Add ½ cup chicken stock, cover the pot, and cook for 10 minutes. When the vegetables are tender, add the wine and simmer until nearly all the liquid evaporates, about 1 to 2 minutes. Stir in the kale, chard, 1 teaspoon salt, and 3 cups of stock. (To make a bisque instead, substitute one cup of milk for one cup of stock. Add the milk at the very end after you have pureed the soup, and be very careful not to boil it.) Cover pot and simmer for 10 to 15 minutes. Add the spinach and cook for another 3 to 5 minutes until the spinach is just wilted. Puree the soup in a blender until it is very smooth. Keep in mind that the hot liquid will expand in the blender, so puree in several batches. Return to the soup pot and thin with a little more stock or water if the soup seems too thick. Heat over low heat until just hot. Serve immediately, sprinkled with Parmesan cheese.

Serves 6–8.

NEW GOURMET GREENS

By Omri Aronow
Chef at Rick and Ann's
Berkeley, California

Spring Spinach Salad

GREENS

2 cups baby spinach
1 hard-boiled egg, sliced
½ cup olives (your favorite kind)

DRESSING

2 red bell peppers
1 clove garlic
½ cup extra-virgin olive oil

1 tablespoon flaxseed oil
2 tablespoons vinegar (sherry vinegar is best)
salt and pepper to taste

Cut the bell peppers into quarters, remove the seeds and white sections, and chop coarsely. Put all of the dressing ingredients into a blender and pulse until the dressing is smooth. Mix the spinach with the dressing. Garnish with egg slices and olives.
Serves 2–4.

Pacific Coast Caesar Salad

1 head of romaine lettuce
2 ounces sardines
3 tablespoons white wine vinegar
1 teaspoon capers
1 teaspoon mustard
½ cup olive oil
2 tablespoons flaxseed oil
salt and pepper to taste
¼ cup grated Parmesan cheese (or your
    favorite hard cheese)
½ cup croutons (optional)

Wash and chop the romaine into bite-sized strips. Put the rest of the ingredients, except the cheese and croutons, into a blender and mix until smooth. Toss the romaine with the dressing from the blender. Garnish with grated cheese and croutons.
Serves 2–4.

Kohav's Tabouli Salad
¼ cup boiling water
¼ cup bulgur wheat
1 tablespoon flaxseed or olive oil
¼ cup lemon juice
½ cup finely chopped mint
1½ cups finely chopped parsley
½ cup finely chopped red bell pepper
1 teaspoon ground coriander seeds
(optional)
salt and pepper to taste
½ cup cucumber slices

In a mixing bowl, pour the boiling water over the bulgar and let it steep for 10 minutes. Add the oil and lemon juice and let the mixture steep for another 15 minutes. Add the mint, parsley, and bell pepper and season with salt and pepper to taste and coriander. Serve with cucumber slices as garnish.
Serves 4.

Midsummer Parsley Soup
2 bunches of parsley, washed and finely
chopped
5 cups boiling water
3 cups soup stock (chicken or vegetable)
2 cups cream (or milk)
2 egg yolks
salt and cayenne pepper to taste
parsley sprig

Blanch the parsley by dipping it into the boiling water for 5 seconds. Discard the water and bring the soup stock to a boil. Add the parsley and simmer gently for 15 minutes until the parsley is very tender. Take the stock and parsley off the burner and let it cool to room temperature. Pour the stock and parsley into a blender and blend, then pour back into a stovetop pot. Add the cream (or milk) and egg yolks and heat gently on low for 3 to 6 minutes, stirring continuously, until the soup thickens slightly (do not boil!). Season to taste with salt and cayenne pepper. Cool in the refrigerator and serve chilled with a sprig of parsley as garnish.

Serves 4.

San Francisco Spinach Soup

2 medium onions, chopped
2 celery ribs, chopped
1 leek, chopped
2 garlic cloves
1 small potato, chopped
1 bay leaf
1 pound spinach (3–4 bunches)
1 quart of stock (chicken or vegetable)
salt and pepper to taste
4 tablespoons sour cream

Bring the stock to a boil and add the onions, celery, leek, garlic, potato, and bay leaf. Simmer for about 30 minutes until all the vegetables are ten-

der (do not boil). Remove the bay leaf and add the spinach. If you are using fresh, rather than frozen, spinach, cook it in the soup until it wilts. Season with salt and pepper to taste. Serve as is for a chunky texture, or puree in a blender. Garnish with 1 tablespoon of sour cream per serving.
Serves 4.

Great Grapefruit Greens
¾ cup grapefruit juice
3 tablespoons mustard
1 tablespoon chopped basil
1 teaspoon minced garlic (optional)
2 cups chopped beet greens
2 cups chopped collard greens
2 cups chopped kale
½ teaspoon ground allspice (optional)
salt and pepper to taste

Add the grapefruit juice, mustard, basil, and garlic to a large pot and bring to a boil. Immediately add the greens and cook until wilted. Season with salt and pepper to taste and allspice.
Serves 4.

Japanese Peanut Chard
2 bunches of Swiss chard, washed
½ cup sliced shiitake mushrooms (or your favorite mushrooms)
3 tablespoons olive oil
½ cup soup stock (chicken or vegetable)

2 tablespoons soy sauce

salt and pepper to taste

¼ cup chopped, roasted peanuts

Cut the stems off the chard and chop them into small cubes. Slice the leaves into 1-to-1½-inch lengths. Sauté the mushrooms and the cubed stems in the olive oil for about 3 to 4 minutes. Add the chard leaves and cook for about 4 more minutes. Add the soup stock and soy sauce and cook until the leaves are tender. Season with salt and pepper to taste and garnish with peanuts.

Serves 4.

Wine Country Salmon with Spinach Sauce

2 quarts water salted with 2 tablespoons salt

1 compressed cup (1–2 bunches) of washed
    spinach

juice of 1 lemon

3 tablespoons olive oil

1 tablespoon flaxseed oil

4 tablespoons ice water

salt and pepper to taste

1 bay leaf (optional)

1 tablespoon crushed fennel seeds (optional)

2 6-ounce salmon filets ½-to-1-inch thick,
    lightly salted

1 cup cooking white wine

4 lemon slices

Drop the spinach into boiling, lightly salted water and cook until very tender but still green. Strain and put in a blender with the lemon juice, oil, and ice water. Blend well and season to taste with salt and pepper. In a pan, bring the wine, bay leaf, and fennel seeds to a boil, immediately reduce to a simmer, and place the salted salmon filets skin side down in the wine. Cover the pan tightly and cook for 4 to 6 minutes. Remove and place on a plate. Top with the spinach sauce and garnish with lemon slices. You may want to serve the salmon with a side of mashed potatoes mixed with the bell pepper dressing from the Spring Spinach Salad recipe.

Serves 2.

Sierra Mountain Stew

1 cup (7-ounce) black beans
2 chicken breasts, cubed
1 tablespoon olive oil
1 large onion, chopped
3 garlic cloves, sliced
3 bunches of spinach (about 2 cups cooked),
    washed and chopped
salt and pepper to taste

Submerge the beans in a pot of unsalted water so that they arc covered by 1 inch of water. Soak them this way overnight, and then move the pot to the stove. Cook the beans, still submerged, until they are tender. Save about ½ a cup of this cooking liquid. In a pan, brown the chicken cubes with olive oil, add the onion, and cook for about 5 minutes until the onion is tender. Add the sliced garlic and cook for 1 more minute. Add the chopped spinach and beans and cook for about 5 more minutes, until the spinach is wilted. If the stew is too dry, add some of the cooking liquid from the beans. Season with salt and pepper to taste.

Serves 2–4.

West Coast Style Alabama Sausage Cakes

10-ounce sausage, sliced and diced (your
   favorite kind)
1 teaspoon olive oil
1 cup collard greens, washed and chopped
1 cup corn kernels (freshly cooked, defrosted,
   or canned)
salt and pepper to taste
2 eggs
1 tablespoon chopped cilantro (optional)
1 teaspoon chili flakes (optional)
½ cup flour
½ cup cornmeal
canola oil for frying

Sauté the sausage with the olive oil. Add the collard greens and cook until they are wilted. Add the corn and season with salt and pepper to taste. Remove from heat and set the mixture in a large bowl. Beat the eggs and then mix them in the bowl with the sausage, greens, cilantro, and chili flakes. When this mixture has cooled, add the flour gradually until the mixture is doughy and kneed it into 4-oz. balls with your fingers. Press the balls into the cornmeal for coating and so they form patties about 1 inch thick. Fry the patties in canola oil on medium to low heat until they are golden. Do not fry too quickly or they will not cook on the inside. Drain on paper towels and serve.

Serves 4.

PART II:

Experiencing AMD

CHAPTER 5

I Am Not Blind: The Shock of AMD

I am not blind. Do not tell me that I am blind. I refuse to be blind. I hate that word.

—Grace Olsen

When I first met Grace Olsen, she was wearing a blue wool dress with pearl buttons. She had her hair in a pretty blond bob, and she held her chin up. At eighty-two, she looked not a day over seventy, and she was fierce. She eyed me unapologetically and observed that she'd been to two other ophthalmologists since she'd been diagnosed with macular degeneration, including her retinal specialist, and none of them had much to say. "My son thinks I should go to the School for the Blind in Kalamazoo," she said evenly, "but I am not blind. Do not tell me that I am blind. I refuse to be blind. I hate that word." No, I agreed, she was not blind and she would not go blind from macular degeneration. But with 20/200 acuity in both eyes, she did have low vision. "You have no idea what this is like," Grace continued, her voice becoming softer. "It's such a shock. You cannot understand unless it happens to you." And then she quietly began to cry.

YOU HAVE NO IDEA WHAT THIS IS LIKE

Grace was right. I have no idea what it's like to have macular degeneration. I am already past sixty, though, my father has advanced macular degeneration, and I have his light blue eyes. Since those are all risk factors, I may know in a few years. But talking right now with Grace, I could not tell her that I really understood. Listening and imagining are not the same as living. This is one of the toughest things facing anyone with macular degeneration. It's an experience that's very hard to convey.

Macula What?

Until the late 1990s, virtually no one had heard of age-related macular degeneration. When we wrote the first edition of this book, there were no other books on the topic and few articles in the newspapers. Of course, ophthalmologists knew it existed, but nobody was talking about it at the dinner table. Those diagnosed with AMD found themselves shocked and disoriented. "Macaroni what?" they'd say, or "Immaculate what?" or "Degeneration what?" Then there was Zelda Grant, who called it the macarena after the Latin American dance tune popular in 1996. Zelda, like most everybody else who'd lost vision from AMD, found her family, friends, and neighbors totally confused. "What is a macular?" everyone wondered. As Zelda said, "It's hard to have something that changes your whole life and no one gets it. They can't even say its name."

Today the name isn't any easier to pronounce, but there is much more attention to macular degeneration in the media and at research centers around the country—and the world—than there was as recently as 1998. There has literally been an explosion of new research on macular degeneration in the medical community. Researchers in the Netherlands, Germany, and Japan have been in the forefront of finding new treatments for AMD in the last four years, along with hundreds of leading physicians and scientists at dozens of universities and hospitals here in the United States. Up to 700,000 Americans develop early-stage AMD every year, and 200,000 lose their central vision to it annually. Macular degeneration affects the citizens of every European country and is now appearing in Asia and South America as well, so the race is on to stop this condition and to develop technologies that restore lost sight. We all know its name now, and we're going to lick it.

IT'S HARD TO SEE IF
IT ISN'T HAPPENING TO YOU

We usually associate vision loss with looking different. We expect people with vision loss to be blind and blind people to have obviously damaged or unfocused eyes. But if you have macular degeneration, you won't look any different to your neighbors, friends, or family. You make proper eye contact with people, just like you always have, so they are unlikely to realize that you can't see them clearly. In familiar surroundings, you probably don't appear to be any less competent or confident than you did ten years ago. You may also be able to do much of what you did before macular degeneration, although it may take two to three times longer. "I used to be able to change a doorknob in ten minutes," Joe Toscano reported. "Now I can still do it, but it takes over an hour. An hour for a doorknob! I'm always worried about how much worse it will get. But the neighbors have no idea. To them I look and act just like the same old Joe."

Because you look and act so much like you always have, even best friends and spouses may find it difficult to remember what you can and can't see. "It's amazing how easily even the people closest to me forget," Dolly Kowalski told me. "My friend Maria and I have dinner together almost every night. Last week we went out to an Italian restaurant and Maria says in a disappointed voice, 'Dolly, you haven't said anything about my new necklace.' I just said, 'Have you lost your mind? I can't see that necklace! I didn't even know you were wearing one!' Maria was very quiet. So I said, 'Pass the dates, please.' Then she said gently, 'They're not dates, Dolly; they're olives.' So I winked at her. I figured they were olives. But honestly! She knows I can't recognize people when they walk into the room. What in the world would possess her to think I could see a little pearl necklace?"

So What Can You See?

To say you have macular degeneration is to say that your central vision is affected, but it doesn't say *how much* it is affected. You may have 20/40 visual acuity or 20/600 or anything in between (see chapter 1 for an explanation of visual acuity measurements).

To say you have macular degeneration also doesn't say *how* your vision is affected. And *how* turns out to matter a great deal. AMD reduces central vision, but it also affects contrast sensitivity, glare sensitivity, and depth perception. All of these factors influence your overall experience of seeing.

It's helpful to understand these factors and be aware of what you can and can't see. It's also very helpful for your friends and family to understand your experience of seeing. But remember that to say that you have macular degeneration, or to say you have a certain visual acuity, doesn't say much about what you can or can't do with your vision. It's true that if you have 20/200 vision you aren't likely to qualify for a driver's license. But driver's licenses are legally regulated according to visual acuity. Most activities in life are not. Don't make the leap between being aware of your vision and labeling yourself with limitations.

Contrast Sensitivity

Low contrast sensitivity explains much of what seems peculiar about vision affected by AMD. For example, most people find it difficult to understand or explain why they can see a two-inch letter in a newspaper headline, but they can't recognize their own grandchildren's faces. Most of their relatives find this confusing, too. Maria fell right into this divide when she went to dinner with Dolly and fished for a compliment on the necklace. Dolly could see the olives on the table after all, so why couldn't she see Maria's necklace?

The answer is that Dolly has low contrast sensitivity. Macular degeneration may decrease contrast sensitivity because it affects the ability of the cone cells to tell similar colors or shades apart. As a result, many people with macular degeneration find it difficult to distinguish between navy blue and brown, or pastel pink and pastel orange. In fact, any object that isn't in sharp contrast to its background may be difficult to see. Black-white contrast combinations are always the best. That's why Dolly can see black olives on a white plate; they have excellent contrast and are therefore much easier to see than a pearl necklace against a white sweater, regardless of the size of the necklace.

Human faces are the worst. They have terrible contrast. No matter what color your skin may be, it's probably all the same color, so the contours of your features blend together. "I have four beautiful little grandchildren," Dolly Kowalski said. "They all look equally beautiful to me. In fact, they all look the same. When they visit me we play the 'Who's Kissing Grandma Now?' game. My daughter says, 'How can they look alike? They have such different features.' But what's a nose or a chin when it's the same color as a forehead?" If we all had either extremely light or extremely dark skin, neon orange eyes and lips, and a contrasting-color nose, we'd be much more visible. Until that happens, macular degeneration may make it easier to see a two-inch-high black letter standing against white paper than to see a grandchild's nose. "They're all my favorites," Dolly said. "I tell them, 'Grandma can't see your pretty smiles, so you have to laugh out loud when you're happy.' So they fall over themselves guffawing. My daughter always comes running in and tries to quiet the ruckus."

Glare Sensitivity

Glare sensitivity also affects many people with macular degeneration. Joe Toscano's experience is typical. "I'm actually not too bothered by contrast, especially since Inez matches up my clothes," Joe said, flipping a fluorescent light switch in his kitchen. "But look! I can hardly open my eyes with this glare. When I'm in someone else's house, I find it difficult to see as much as I usually can if they have fluorescent lighting or if the room is flooded with sunlight. I carry a pair of light yellow NOIR sunglasses to cut the glare indoors. My old friend Tony says to me, 'Hey, Joe! What are you doing wearing those goggles inside?' I say, 'Hey, Tony, do you want to play cards or not? No, goggles, no cards. You should wear them, too; they'd make you look better.' Tony just smiles. We've been giving each other a hard time for seventy years. We met in grade school. How about that?"

Depth Perception

Buddy Burmester doesn't notice glare as much as Joe but does have poor depth perception. Poor depth perception may occur when one eye is more affected by AMD than the other, throwing the two out of sync. It may also result from low contrast sensitivity. Contrast sensitivity enhances our depth perception because we use variations in shades and sharp lines to perceive three-dimensional objects. "Have you ever seen a coin at the bottom of a pool, dived for it, and found that it's not where you expected it to be? That's macular degeneration for me," Buddy Burmester said. "It's like living with permanent pool vision. I can't tell you how many times I've reached for a soda can and it's not exactly where I think it is. It's such a difficult experience to convey to anyone else. It's just a difficult experience, period. I'm not even used to it yet."

One of the most frustrating consequences of poor depth perception is that it may make walking in unfamiliar places more precarious. Since walking is important for transportation and exercise, if you have poor depth perception consider using a walking cane for stability or walk with a friend. Explore other forms of physical activity and exercise, such as riding a stationary bicycle, swimming, pool running, weight lifting, gentle stretching classes, or relaxation yoga. Above all, try not to let poor depth perception contribute to isolation and lower activity levels.

THE SHOCK OF DISCOVERING AMD

For some people, macular degeneration comes on gradually, as it did for Sam Weinberg, whose dry AMD progressed very slowly for fifteen years. For others, like Zelda Grant, macular degeneration comes in waves. Initially Zelda was diagnosed with dry macular degeneration and she experienced only minor vision loss in one eye. Three years later, Zelda was at a local conference. As she looked over the presentation schedule posted on a board in the lobby, she reached up and rubbed one eye. To Zelda's shock, the presentation schedule disappeared. She went immediately to her doctor and discovered that she had developed wet macular degeneration. Like Zelda, Grace Olsen also experienced macular degeneration as a sudden, unexpected shock.

Shock Is Not Just Surprise

Feeling shocked can be traumatic itself, above and beyond the actual life change or loss we sustain from the event that shocked us. When we are shocked by a sudden life-threatening or life-changing event, we are more than surprised by something negative. We are hit with a feeling of powerlessness to stop what is happening to us. To a large degree, our sense of security in the world is predicated on our faith that we can determine our present and our future and that we have options. Of course, we can and we do. But shock throws that faith into question. Feeling shocked without hearing about options and paths for action can exacerbate both the shock and the original problem, eventually contributing to depression. To counter shock, it's very important to seek support and visual rehabilitation as soon as you find out about your condition. Unfortunately, many people who have macular degeneration aren't told about resources and rehabilitation programs in their area. They may have received little attention when they were diagnosed. This was Grace Olsen's experience. If this was your experience, too, it's never too late. Seek support now (see appendix A to find a visual rehabilitation program in your area). Like Grace you may still have residual feelings of shock. You may wonder why it happened the way it did.

GRACE OLSEN'S STORY

It happened in the summer of 1997. In June, I bought a beautiful gray Lincoln my husband would have loved. It reminded me so much of him. I drove myself up to Traverse City for the Fourth of July. The humidity was terrible. And the road signs seemed so far away, as if I were looking at them through smoke. I thought it was the heat—waves of hot air rising from the cement. I remember singing "Fly Me to the Moon" and squinting at road signs.

At lunch that Sunday, my sister-in-law Edie leaned in to my ear. "Pass the salt!" she whispered loudly. "It's right there; what's the matter with you?" I never liked Edie. She's so abrupt. But the salt *was* sitting right in front of me. Plain as day. I just didn't see it. When I drove home I noticed that the road signs still seemed hazy. I kept thinking, I must need new glasses. So I went to my ophthalmologist the very next week.

"You have to see a retinal specialist," he said. He didn't sound urgent, just very matter-of-fact. The next Tuesday at nine A.M., I went to see the retinal specialist.

"Well," he said, all upbeat, "you've got macular degeneration. You have some irreversible vision loss, but most importantly, you need laser surgery right now to prevent additional loss. Can someone else drive you home?"

I just stared at him. *"What?"* was all I could say. I felt like I was hearing him through twelve feet of water. He kept talking, but I don't think I heard a word he said after "irreversible vision loss."

My mind just froze on those words. I was
so shocked.

After laser surgery I think my vision
was actually worse in my left eye.
Several days later, I saw the specialist
again. He seemed pleased.

"They're fine," he announced, "I
think we've got it checked."

"Checked?" I said. "What about my
vision? What happened to my vision?"

He didn't seem concerned. "That's to
be expected," he said. "Hopefully you'll
still keep some of your vision this way.
Just stop driving. You won't go blind
from this, so you'll be okay." He patted
me on the arm, and out he went. Just
like that. Just like he was telling me
Hudson's department store was having a
summer sale on whites. With that much
feeling.

But how am I going to be okay if I
stop driving? I live in the metro Detroit
area. You can't do anything without
driving. All my friends live off different
freeway exits. Do you realize that I'd
have to walk two miles on roads without
sidewalks where people are driving forty-
five miles an hour *and* cross two six-lane
intersections in order to get a carton of
milk? How could he tell me I'm going to
be fine and just walk out? How could he?

Shooting the Messenger?

Not everyone has Grace's experience. Many people feel very supported and encouraged by their doctors, especially when their doctors give them information about visual rehabilitation and support groups. But many people do have Grace's experience. When Edina Williams, a polite, petite woman in her eighties, heard Grace's story she said, "Yep. I know what she's talking about. I tell you, if I could drive my car just one more time, I'd use it to run my doctor over." Gentle Dolly Kowalski, of all people, agreed, except that she recollected a shotgun her mother once used on a troublesome man back in 1922 on their farm in rural Indiana. It was very effective. Zelda Grant had another idea: "I'd give him macular degeneration for just one week and see whether he still wants to compare it to the challenges of handling age-related hair loss." What's going on here to provoke this private backlash in so many people? Is it a case of shooting the messenger?

No one wants to hear that they have AMD or irreversible vision loss, but that's not what sets Dolly to thinking about her mother's shotgun. There are actually two problems at hand. The first is a communication problem. While most doctors went into the field because they care about people, and they work very hard to fix their patients' medical conditions, that doesn't mean they know how to communicate effectively. The second problem is one of omission. Too many eye doctors are unaware of the existence of visual rehabilitation and their patients' need for it. They do not realize that they are actually failing to uphold the Hippocratic oath to do no harm when they say, "There's nothing that can be done," and walk out of the room without making any referrals or providing information. A neurologist wouldn't dream of walking away from a patient who could no longer use an arm as the result of a stroke without referring him or her to occupational therapy. So why do some eye doctors leave the room without saying a word?

Why Doctors Can Be Abrupt

In most medical programs, doctors are trained under very stressful work conditions with long hours and little consideration for their own physical, emotional, or personal lives. They must learn to ignore these things for themselves, focus on problem solving, and move quickly. Their achievements are measured by how well they fix the physical problem they were trained to fix, not by how well they related to their patients or by how well they understand the implications of the problem for their patients' lives. When doctors are faced with a problem that they cannot really fix, like macular degeneration, they are faced with their own limitations. And they don't always know how to handle it sensitively.

As a matter of fact, doctors are by far my worst patients at our low-vision rehabilitation program. Although this information may not be particularly comforting, you can rest assured that the more abrupt doctors are, the less likely they are to handle vision loss well if it happens to them. Doctors' take-charge attitude often runs them right into the ground when they get macular degeneration. They have feared vision loss and fought it all their lives by seeking to control it. As you know better than anyone, if there's one thing that macular degeneration takes away from us, it's the ability to conquer by controlling. The people who handle AMD successfully are not the hard-charging executives or the General Patton types. They're the folks with a sense of humor, an abiding faith, and an ability to see the humanity in themselves and others regardless of their vision. They're the folks with a willingness to be flexible, to find other ways to direct their lives rather than by demanding precision and efficiency from everyone and everything around them.

Doctors who communicate well and offer their patients empathy, guidance, and options had to learn how to do that on their own or were lucky enough to have supportive mentors. This is true even in specialties that often deal with death or conditions that bring major life changes. Twelve years ago, my mother was admitted to a hospital near my parents' home with minor chest pain. The staff assured us that she was fine, but she stayed overnight for tests. Sometime in the early morning she suffered a massive heart attack. My father and I waited anxiously at the hospital for news. Eventually, a senior resident came out, stiffened, and blurted, "The code blue was unsuccessful." My father nodded gravely, stood up, and said, "Well, is she awake now? When can I see her?" The young doctor looked stunned. He had no idea what to say next. He had no idea how to tell my father that his beloved wife of fifty-three years had just died. He had used the only language he was taught, which is what many doctors do.

Your Doctor Should Refer You to Visual Rehabilitation

Family practitioners often don't refer their patients to visual rehabilitation because they assume the ophthalmologist will do it—after all, macular degeneration is an eye condition. But many ophthalmologists are not familiar with programs in their area; they may not even realize such programs exist, since visual rehabilitation is not a standard part of ophthalmology training and the field is so new in medicine. Until recently, visual rehabilitation programs were designed almost exclusively for fully blind children or young adults; there were very few programs that addressed the needs and skills of seniors with partial vision loss. That's changing.

Today Medicare covers visual rehabilitation

for macular degeneration in all fifty states, and we look forward to new programs developing in the near future. State commissions for the blind are revising their program offerings to include seniors. Visual rehabilitation programs are opening their doors around the country, and occupational therapy schools are realizing that we need occupational therapists who can work with people who have macular degeneration, too. There's a great effort nationwide to educate doctors about these programs and the importance of visual rehabilitation. Until the word is out, though, you may have to take matters into your own hands.

To find rehabilitation programs in your area, follow the guide in appendix A. Keep in mind that programs vary in quality and scope, so it's best to check out all of your options. In some areas of the country, programs are not covered by insurance or are not available. This was one of the biggest reasons that we wrote this book: so that it could serve as your own personal visual rehabilitation program or as a supplement to one in your area. In part III of this book you'll find a complete home version of our program here in Michigan.

The Importance of Early Visual Rehabilitation

The time to start visual rehabilitation is now—as soon as you begin to experience any vision loss at all. Some programs will only accept participants with vision of 20/70 or less or, in some cases, 20/200 or less in their better eye. But we know that the earlier you start visual rehabilitation the better off you will be. This does not mean giving up on your sight or future treatments. You can still focus on keeping your eyes healthy and learn the lifesaving principles of visual rehabilitation at the same time. When it comes to living with macular degeneration, the more you know, the stronger you will be. If you do not qualify for a program in your area, you can still begin visual rehabilitation using part III of this book.

How Shock Interrupts Understanding

Often, when doctors do talk, we can't hear them. Just as Grace said that she didn't hear anything her doctor said after he told her she had "irreversible vision loss," it's often difficult for anyone to assimilate anything said after a shock. Our minds protect us emotionally by tuning out information that overwhelms us. Sometimes we don't even realize we've tuned out. We just don't remember that anything was said. I often find myself repeating information upon request, knowing that it's natural for people to have difficulty digesting it all at once. It's also easy to forget questions while you're at your doctor's office. Try the following five tips for talking with your doctor and getting the most out of your appointment.

FIVE TIPS FOR TALKING WITH YOUR DOCTOR

1. Brainstorm your questions before your appointment, write them down with a black felt-tipped pen, and take them with you.

2. Take a friend or family member along so there are two sets of ears listening in the room.

3. If your doctor's explanations aren't easily understandable, ask for an assistant in the office who can explain in clear detail and answer questions.

4. Ask your doctor for a referral to a rehabilitation program and support group in your area.

5. Don't take it personally if your doctor isn't supportive or seems rushed. It is not a reflection of your condition or your potential.

BEYOND SHOCK: ZELDA'S AND SAM'S EXPERIENCES

Just as people have different experiences of vision loss with macular degeneration, they also have different experiences of coping. We left Grace at a moment of crisis. After her diagnosis, she felt so overwhelmed with the enormity of losing her driver's license, with fears of blindness, and with the absence of information or assistance that she struggled with depression for two years. Grace's depression lifted when she moved to a socially active senior community, came to visual rehabilitation, received some counseling, and joined a support group. "For a time, macular degeneration took my life away," Grace reflected. "Now I've started a new one." As Judy Prevost puts in her on-line memoir, "Macular degeneration can either hurl us into an unforgiving depression or teach us new ways of seeing and feeling that we have never experienced before." Like Grace, Zelda Grant faced shock, but Zelda's fiery personality and her doctor's support made the experience different for her. Sam Weinberg, however, never really felt shocked. He was diagnosed with dry macular degeneration fifteen years ago, and his vision loss progressed very slowly, giving Sam plenty of time to adjust. Macular degeneration has, however, caused Sam to question his approach to life. He has worked to cultivate his sense of humor, which has helped him adjust to macular degeneration.

ZELDA GRANT'S STORY

The day my doctor told me that I had low vision from macular degeneration, I came home and smashed every dish in the house. All twelve place settings, two platters, and a cake plate. They were white china with little blue flowers that looked like little squiggly bugs to me. At the time, I was crying and screaming and smashing. There were chips everywhere; the kitchen floor was a mess.

When I was done, all I had left were a half-dozen navy blue plastic bowls and a few coffee mugs, but I saved my life. If I hadn't smashed those dishes I'd be an angry woman with a pretty dining room setting that I couldn't really see anyway. I was angry for a long time as it was, and I sometimes still am, but smashing those dishes was a turning point, a declaration. I am going to live, and worrying about little blue flower bugs on my plates is not a part of living anymore.

Besides, if I hadn't smashed those plates it never would have occurred to me to get brightly colored plastic daily dishes that are easier to see and harder to break. The navy blue bowls gave me that idea. On a white tablecloth, they are much more visible than white china ever could be.

So after I cleaned up my kitchen, I went through the information packet my doctor gave me, and began to make some phone calls. I called a rehabilitation program in my area and I said, "Hello. My name is Zelda Grant. I want an appointment, and I want to know how I'm going to keep reading." And then I called the neighborhood community center and said, "Hello. My name is Zelda Grant. I have low vision and I think I have a lot of energy. I need an exercise class." And then I called the support group listed in my information packet, and I said, "Hello. My name is Zelda Grant. What do you people talk about anyway?" I didn't bank on much to start with, but the more calls I made, and the more people I talked to, the easier it was to get help, and to do the things I wanted to do.

You know, there are many people with inspiring approaches to life. I recently heard a quote from a paraplegic man named Mark Wellman who climbed a mountain at Yosemite National Park. Can you imagine climbing a mountain without using your legs? He says, "You have a dream and you know the only way that dream is going to happen is if you do it . . . even if it's six inches at a time."

Now that's even a little much for me. I have a simpler motto. I just say, no matter who you are, if you stop trying you're dead. You just forgot to lie down.

SAM WEINBERG'S STORY

I first learned I had dry macular degeneration fifteen years ago. My doctor said, "Sam, you've got drusen here, but just a very slight amount of vision loss." I immediately thought, My God, what's going to happen to my law practice? I have a small-town private practice, mostly estate planning and compensation. I really worried that as soon as everyone knew, they'd decide they didn't want a visually impaired attorney. So I did everything I could to camouflage my low vision. I didn't even tell Rachel initially. I pretended I could see everything. I stayed up late at night using a magnifier and a bright desk lamp to read small-print documents and memorize them, so I could quote them verbatim and I wouldn't have to refer to papers during meetings. When new clients came, I called my secretary into

the office and asked her to take detailed
notes, type them, and print them in large
font, so I wouldn't have to take notes
myself. I stopped trying to read tiny price
labels in the grocery store. I just took a
lot of money with me and paid whatever
the total came out to be. Rachel got
suspicious pretty quickly. One day she
eyed me and said, "You used to love
coupons. What happened?"

After a few years, I just couldn't
keep it a secret any longer, especially
when my vision got worse. Rachel said,
"Sam, they know you. They know you're
a good lawyer. You're still a good
lawyer." I didn't believe her at first, but
she was right. My regular clients have
been really loyal. They consult with me
about ongoing issues, and bring me new
cases. I also do a fair amount of
consulting to younger attorneys,
especially in the compensation field,
since I know so much at this point. I
work forty hours a week. And I spend a
lot of time reading relevant journals and
keeping up on the field. I have CCTV's
[closed-circuit TVs] for my office and my
home, I have big-print software for my
computer, and a large monitor. I use
tape recorders for important meetings
and depositions, I use floodlights in my

office, and I write everything with black felt-tip pens. My secretary has gotten really adept at a low-vision legal practice.

Sometimes I think Rachel would prefer it if I weren't working so hard. Actually, I've been thinking about cutting back because I'd like to spend more time with my violin. When I was young, I wanted to be a professional musician, but it didn't seem financially feasible. I figure now's my chance to play all the time!

Low vision has challenged me to be less earnest. I'm an overachiever, and that's gotten me far in life. But sometimes I forget to have a good time. So I've really tried to strengthen my sense of humor, and not take it all too seriously. Rachel keeps me on my toes. We went to a big party last week. Rachel wore a pair of distinctive black-and-white patent-leather shoes. She disappeared into the crowd, so I went looking for her shoes. When I thought I'd found them, I leaned over, puckered up, and whispered, "Are you my wife?"

This woman jumped six inches, and huffed, "I certainly hope not!"

"Too bad," I said, "You don't know what you're missing!"

I Am Not Blind

At the same party, I ate dry cat food.
It was sitting in a bowl on the kitchen
counter looking just like mixed nuts and
pretzels. Rachel said, "Sam! What am I
going to do with you?" And we laughed
so hard we had tears in our eyes.

CHAPTER 6

With the Heart
One Sees Rightly:
Living Fully with AMD

It is with the heart that one sees rightly; what is essential is invisible to the eye.
—Antoine de Saint-Exupéry
The Little Prince

I have met many people in the last few years whose courage matches their despair, whose hearts are still hopeful, people who are both defiant and defeated, angry and optimistic, fearful and faithful. As Bette Davis put it, "Growing old ain't for sissies." And neither is macular degeneration. But seniors are hardly sissies. If you are in your nineties, by the time you were half your age you had experienced two world wars and the greatest depression in the history of this country. If you are in your eighties, you may barely remember World War I, but you spent your teen years during the Depression and your young adulthood in World War II. If you are in your seventies, you missed World War I entirely, you just made World War II, and then you got to send your son to Vietnam. You grew up without Social Security, penicillin, civil rights movement, Title IX, Alcoholics Anonymous, Dr. Spock, and permanent press, and that's not easy. If you are in your sixties and have just discovered, on the eve of your retirement, that you are losing your vision, with twenty or thirty years of living ahead of you, that's not easy, either.

You have probably already experienced profound losses in your life, but losing vision is a new kind of loss. Unlike deaths, accidents, or serious illnesses, AMD comes quietly, often without public recognition, certainly without flowers or phone calls. It doesn't seem very dramatic until it happens to you. As Buddy Burmester said, "You wouldn't believe how often you use your eyes every day for everything. But it's not just that I can't see what I want to see. It affects my sense of control over my life, and my confidence with other people. It affects everything. I guess I assumed my eyes would always be there for me."

Since vision loss is a new kind of loss, it raises new issues and requires new coping skills that may be unfamiliar to you. They include: expressing your feelings, addressing depression, joining the macular degeneration community, exercising for better health, taking risks, and starting visual rehabilitation.

EXPRESSING YOUR FEELINGS

For many people, losing vision is like losing a loved one. You may have very strong feelings about your vision loss: feelings of anger, frustration, fear, regret, embarrassment, or grief. Vision loss deserves grieving and acknowledgment. You don't have to smash plates like Zelda Grant, but give yourself permission to feel strongly and permission to express your feelings. Expressing your feelings means identifying how you feel and sharing your feelings in all of their depth and richness with a friend, family member, religious adviser, or counselor. Some people even share their feelings with their pets. Others turn to a patron saint. Turn to someone with whom you feel comfortable, someone who will listen supportively and acknowledge your feelings.

Just as there are many different people to whom you may turn, there are also many different ways of expressing your feelings. Expressing your feelings may mean crying, screaming, whispering, writing, dancing, walking, just plain old talking, or punching a pillow. Expressing your feelings may also be a process that unfolds over time and through many conversations. Zelda didn't accept having low vision in one afternoon. I doubt anyone does. Whatever you do, though, don't bottle yourself up and tell yourself that there's no reason to have feelings at all.

"Express your feelings" may be advice that

makes sense to you, but it may not. If you are over sixty-five, you were probably raised to be polite and to keep private matters private. Women in senior generations were taught to make others comfortable whenever possible. Men were taught that feelings are a sign of weakness. And everyone was taught to get tough and pull themselves up by the bootstraps. Feelings weren't even really a topic of public conversation until the baby boomers became the Me generation. Before 1965, feelings were things you had about your first crush. Having too many of them wasn't generally considered a good idea. They might get in the way of meeting your responsibilities at work or at home. But the fact that you don't show your feelings doesn't mean you don't have them. And if you don't acknowledge them, they may weigh heavily on you or they may erupt in other areas of your life, or you may spend so much energy keeping them in check that you aren't really free to feel fully alive or face the future.

Pulling Yourself Up by the Bootstraps

So does expressing your feelings mean you shouldn't pull yourself up by the bootstraps? Is bootstrapping a thing of the past? Absolutely not. It's still a good thing. But today's bootstrapping is different from yesterday's. Pulling yourself up by the bootstraps used to mean doing it all alone. It used to mean having as few needs and as few feelings as possible. It used to mean being carefully dignified and keeping a stiff upper lip. It used to mean saving your money to buy white gloves for Sundays or for shopping downtown. But the world has changed in the last thirty-five years. Now we wear sweatpants to the airport and the doctor's office, neighbors and friends talk openly about coping with breast cancer or alcoholism, and strangers reveal their private lives on national television. As a society, we've taken off the white gloves. But as individuals, we often keep them close at hand. We still cling to the idea that coping well means being quiet and dignity means doing things properly the first time. But that's not true, and it's an idea that isn't doing us any favors.

Redefining Bootstrapping

Zelda Grant was bootstrapping when she had a screaming fit in her kitchen and smashed all her plates. She was bootstrapping when she called for a visual rehabilitation appointment and when she called her neighborhood club to enroll in an exercise class. And she was bootstrapping when she called her local low-vision support group and said, "Hello. My name is Zelda Grant. What do you people talk about anyway?" She may not be winning any points for tact or diplomacy, but as a bootstrapper she's a champion. Bootstrapping today means having feelings, figuring out what they are, and expressing them. Bootstrapping today means having needs, figuring out what they are, and getting them met. Bootstrapping today means asking for the support you need and learning the skills that will enable you to do as much as you can.

Most important, though, bootstrapping today means putting the white gloves away. It means taking the risk that you won't do it properly the first time, that you won't avoid every spill, that you won't always look absolutely perfect. And it means realizing that that's okay. Bootstrapping means putting on your finest clothes for a dinner party and chuckling when you realize you've served paper towels in the tossed salad. Because the truth is that nobody really minds. People like you for you, not for what you can see. Bootstrapping means enjoying their company and realizing that the greatest dignity of all comes from just living.

DEPRESSION AND AMD

Many people who lose vision go through a short period of mild depression as they grieve their loss and adjust their lives. But many others experience prolonged periods of depression that are unhealthy for the body and spirit. We know a great deal more about depression than we did twenty or thirty years ago. We know that it's not a sign of weakness, laziness, or moral failure. We know that depression happens to people who have no other psychological difficulties. We know that depression can happen to you later in life even if you've never been depressed before. And we know that depression is very common among people with low vision. There is nothing shameful about it, but there is something very tragic about living with depression without getting help.

Common Symptoms of Depression

Consider the following list and ask yourself whether or not any of these symptoms are familiar:

- Frequently feeling apathetic or unmotivated

- Frequently feeling agitated, empty, or numb

- Frequently feeling pessimistic or negative about yourself

- Withdrawing socially

- Insomnia or hypersomnia (sleeping too little or too much)

- Losing or gaining more than 5 percent of your body weight in a month

- Noticeable decrease in energy

- Unexplained episodes of crying, emotional swings, or outbursts

- Frequently focusing on regrets

What Causes Depression with Macular Degeneration?

Depression with macular degeneration may arise from deep feelings of rage, grief, frustration, loneliness, from prolonged inactivity or boredom, from losing faith or hope, from self-judgment, fearing the future, or feeling out of control. One of the strongest findings about depression with macular degeneration, strangely enough, is that it is not related to the amount of vision you lose. There are people with very mild vision loss who experience very serious depression and people with very serious vision loss who experience little depression at all. Why? It turns out that whether or not you experience depression depends on a number of factors that are unique to each of us. Some people are genetically predisposed to depression. Your diet and exercise patterns also make a difference, especially if you are sensitive to sugar or alcohol. Function is a huge factor. The more you are able to do with low vision, the less likely you are to become depressed or stay depressed. That's one of the reasons that visual rehabilitation is so important. The good news about rehabilitation is that what you can do is not necessarily determined by how much you can see, as counterintuitive as this sounds. Yes, you may not be able to do everything—or even many things—the same way, but there are almost always alternatives. Seeking alternatives is a powerful antidote to depression, the wooden stake to its Draculean presence. The earlier and more assertively you seek alternatives for doing the things you'd like to do, the narrower the window of opportunity long-term depression has to take hold.

A Word on Driving

If you live in a car-centered area, like most suburban communities, and you lose your driver's license, you may be at greater risk of depression. Cars are often central to our lives. It's beyond inconvenient not to be able to drive—it can rob us of our spontaneity, and it can be discouraging and isolating. As John Patrick Reynolds put it bluntly, "You might as well shoot me. Why do I want to live if I can't drive?" If you share John's feeling, or even a fraction of it, it's essential to seek out alternatives to driving in your area. See chapter 13, "Saving Sight on the Road: Driving, Alternatives, and Traveling," for suggestions. If you are considering relocating, choose a home within an accessible distance of shops, your friends, and your places of work, volunteering, and worship. Homes near bus or rail stops, near lighted crosswalks, with good sidewalks, and within an easy walk of town are ideal. Senior communities with free transit services are also ideal. Do not choose a place that will isolate you.

Why You Can't Always Strong-Arm Your Way Out

Many seniors make the mistake of thinking they should strong-arm their way out of depression. Worse, they think that if they can't strong-arm their way out, there's something wrong with them. Worst of all, they think they just have to live with it. People often come to my office to talk about their vision. They say, "Well, I guess I just have to make the best of it," then set their jaws and look away. Sometimes the gentlest people cry, and sometimes the proudest people cry, as Grace Olsen did. They don't mean they have to make the best of low vision. They mean they have to make the best of being *depressed* with low vision. But depression is not something you want to put up with and embrace as a partner in life. It's bad for your physical health, your emotional health, and your spirit. Depression can also negatively affect your relationships with other people and strain your marriage. Don't decide that you just have to make the best of depression. And don't camouflage it.

There are two reasons why you may not be able to strong-arm your way out of depression, and neither of them has anything to do with being weak. First, depression is a real physiological condition, not just a mind-set or a bad attitude. Research suggests that stressful situations and significant losses in our lives affect the production and regulation of chemicals in our brains that influence our emotional state and our immune system. Once you are depressed, you may remain depressed if you do not receive professional help and take direct action, because the balance of chemicals in your brain may actually promote your depression or at least sustain it. Second, if your depression was triggered by loneliness, isolation, or inactivity, it is unlikely to lift from thinking alone. You need to address the root of the problem.

Treating Depression

The more you do, the better. The first thing you should do, however, is talk to your doctor. Then act on the following suggestions with his or her advice:

- Ask your doctor about antidepressant medications and alternatives, like St. John's Wort, a mild herbal remedy popular in Europe. St. John's Wort has fewer side effects than medications and may be less expensive, but it also may affect your blood pressure.

- If you are sensitive to sugar, ask your doctor about switching to a *balanced* protein-based diet designed to keep your blood sugar levels stable.

- Begin a regular routine of physical exercise (see the suggestions under "Live Through Exercise"). Exercise acts on our brain chemicals to stabilize our moods and has been shown to be an effective antidote for mild to moderate depression in many people.

- Attend a visual rehabilitation program in your area (see appendix A for a guide to finding one) and follow the program in part III of this book.

- Cultivate activities, interests, and friends. Making new friends may seem difficult, especially if you've had the same friends for decades and you're out of practice, and low vision doesn't make it easier. But when friends move or pass away or when your spouse dies, it's really important to reconnect with others. And you can do it. Loneliness and inactivity are not good for you, and you must do whatever you can to avoid them. Consider moving to an active senior center if there is no one to socialize with and not much to do in your area.

- Seek alternatives for getting around town (see chapter 13).

- Seek professional counseling, especially counseling that complements your visual rehabilitation by understanding your feelings and encouraging your skills.

- Join a support group. If you live with someone who has low vision and you are experiencing depression yourself, you need to join a support group, too.

YOU ARE IN GOOD COMPANY: THE AMD COMMUNITY

The macular degeneration community in the United States has millions of members. If you have macular degeneration, you are in good company. You may be sixty or you may be one hundred. You may be a homemaker, small business owner, journalist, national master's swimmer, retired trucker, engineer, parent, grandparent, or great-grandparent, a famous painter like Georgia O'Keeffe, an actress like Phyllis Diller, or a former First Lady like Lady Bird Johnson. You may have just discovered that you have macular degeneration, or you may have been living with it for decades. Whoever you are and whatever your vision, there are many, many people in the United States who share this condition with you. They're right in your neighborhood, and they're all across the country, too.

Memoirs by People with Vision Loss

In the last few years, people with macular degeneration and vision loss from other eye conditions have begun to write about their experiences, reaching out to others with low vision and telling the world the way it is. Journalist Henry Grunwald published his memoir, *Twilight: Losing Sight, Gaining Insight,* about his experience with macular degeneration and poet Stephen Kuusisto published his collection of poems, *Only Bread, Only Light,* and his autobiography, *Planet of the Blind,* about his experience of partial blindness since childhood. Activist and writer Georgina Kleege wrote *Sight Unseen,* a strong critique of our understandings of vision and vision loss, and John Hull wrote *Touching the Rock,* a moving account of his experience of total blindness in midlife. Some old favorites are also still in print, including Frances Lief Neer's edited volume of stories and reflections by people with macular degeneration, *Perceiving the Elephant.* See appendix A for a complete bibliography.

Macular Degeneration Organizations

There are three major associations founded by and for people with macular degeneration: AMD, MDI, and MDP.

The Association for Macular Diseases (AMD) started twenty years ago as a support group in New York City. Today AMD has thousands of members nationwide. Under the leadership of Nikolai Stevenson, who gives wonderful speeches around the country about his experience with macular degeneration and low vision, AMD publishes a large-print quarterly newsletter with tips and research updates and provides other services. You can join AMD by calling 212-605-3719 or visiting www.macula.org.

Tom Perski, M.A., who has low vision from Stargardt's disease, the juvenile form of macular degeneration, founded Macular Degeneration International (MDI) in Tucson in 1991 for people with Stargardt's and age-related macular degeneration. MDI has thousands of members worldwide and offers a large-print biannual news journal with research updates, programs at their Tucson facility, and free seminars around the country. You can join MDI by calling 800-393-7634 or visiting www.maculardegeneration.org.

The Macular Degeneration Partnership (MDP), a Los Angeles coalition of physicians, patients, and families, works to educate doctors about visual rehabilitation. MDP offers a monthly on-line newsletter and E-mail subscription service, AMD Update and will also answer any questions you may have after visiting their Web site information pages at www.amd.org or listening to their recorded information at 888-430-9898, where you can also leave a message.

AMD Internet Communities

If you have Internet access, join MD Support at www.mdsupport.org, a vibrant on-line community founded by Dan Roberts in Kansas City, Missouri, who also has low vision from a macular condition. MD Support has hundreds of members across North America and England and offers timely information and the kind of understanding that others can give only after they've been there themselves. Have a computer software question? Heard a new report on submacular surgery? Harried by worries about financial security? Need tips for handling colleagues or clients? Feeling like you're not going to make it through this? Found new ways to do something? Fallen in love again? Started a new life? Share it with MD Support through their E-mail list group or Internet message board. "It's like having a huge worldwide staff," says Roberts. "Everyone's sharing support and information, working for the benefit of everyone else and for themselves, too. There's no more powerful way to feel good about yourself and your life than to help others."

There are also several excellent personal sites posted by people with macular degeneration (see appendix A for Web addresses). Judy Prevost of Quebec, an active member and volunteer for MD Support, hosts "Judy's Jolts of Hope," a searingly honest, inspiring memoir of her experience of sudden vision loss from wet AMD. Judy expresses the experience of so many people with AMD and shares with us the jolts—the tips, thoughts, and turning points—that moved her from despair to hope. Fellow Canadians Brian

Herron of Ontario and Linda Olsen of British Columbia (no relation to Grace Olsen) also have great sites. I recently contacted Linda about her experience with macular degeneration and I wanted to share her words with you.

LINDA OLSEN'S STORY

For an otherwise independent baby boomer bachelor or bachelorette like me, everything seems impossible when vision loss happens. With nobody else around to help pull out a splinter, set the alarm clock, or find lost keys, the impossible stretches out forever. I was an executive assistant and 90 percent of my job was reading. I remember panicking about having to learn a whole new skill— reading with low vision—and wondering how I would be able to afford the rent for my apartment on the kind of job I could get if I lost this one. I imagined throwing myself on my sister's generosity, living in her basement, and selling pencils on the street corner to contribute to the household expenses.

It was after I discovered MD Support, and especially after traveling to New York City to meet a bunch of them a couple years ago, that my view changed. I realized that even those with the worst vision were doing very interesting and important things, far more interesting and important than anything I was doing before I lost my vision. I slipped out of my fearful state then and got on with my life in a more active and less self-conscious manner.

In the three years since my introduction to macular degeneration, I've learned to read with low vision, found a new executive assistant job, fallen in love, moved to a new home, redecorated it, and traveled to Europe. I've also taken on a new sideline as a Homestay Mom and coach to English language students. As MD Support member Dave Pearce says, "There is life after MD!" I guess I'm proving him right, because my life has been getting better ever since. Who would have thought it possible? But it was possible only when I realized it wasn't just my story. I wasn't really alone. I was facing an experience that lots of others are facing, too. It was only when I talked with them that everything became possible.

Join a Support Group

As Linda's story attests, joining a support group is a very powerful way to be a part of your community. It can also be a great experience. Some people assume that support groups are only for people with talkative personalities or those who can't cope on their own. But that's not true. Support groups are for everyone. Lots of people who don't have low vision have a support group; they just don't call it that. For example, the Rotary Club, the Lions Club, the chamber of commerce, and small business associations are all support groups. They are places to share a common experience, get advice and tips, network and meet others, do some good for the community, and avoid having to reinvent the wheel on your own. Call your local visual rehabilitation program for support group information (see appendix A to find a program nearby) or join MD Support.

Start Your Own

If there is no support group in your area, it doesn't mean that there aren't any seniors with low vision in your area; it just means that no one is getting the benefit of a support group. Everyone is reinventing the wheel all by themselves and feeling very alone doing it. Why not start a group? Use the following suggestions as a handy guideline:

- To find members, ask your clergy to announce a new support group, publish an announcement in the newsletter or weekly bulletin, or distribute flyers in big print at local places of worship and senior centers. Include your phone number so people can call and ask questions.

- Call your local paper and ask them to interview you about living with macular degeneration and profile your efforts to start a support group. Tell them there are probably thousands of other people living with low vision in the community.

- Ask your local senior or community center or house of worship for free meeting space. Collect public transportation information for that location and consider arranging for shared rides or taxis for members.

- At your first meeting, decide on regular meeting times, topics of interest, and discussion format. You can simply share recent experiences or use sections of this book as a framework for discussions by reading passages aloud.

- Set some basic ground rules as a group. The National Association for the Visually Handicapped (NAVH) recommends a few and offers a large-print booklet on how to start a support group (see appendix C under low-vision catalogs):

— Always introduce everyone in the room each week. Introduce yourself if you arrive late.

— Avoid whispering. Speak clearly enough so everyone can hear. If you can't hear someone else clearly, ask them to speak up.

— Keep a confidentiality rule about discussions of private matters, such as relationships with spouses. Everything said in the group stays in the group.

THE STORIES WE HEAR AND THE STORIES WE TELL

New books and audiotapes that talk to, for, or about seniors seem to arrive on the bookstore shelves in a steady stream. There are new memoirs, new philosophies, such as that in Rabbi Salman Schachter-Shalomi's *From Age-ing to Sage-ing: A Profound New Vision of Growing Older*, and new reports on health, like *Successful Aging: The MacArthur Foundation Study*. Although each book takes a different approach, they all tell the same truth: that being a senior is a stage of life as important as every other stage. Seniors are a growing part of American society. Even though we may not have the bodies we used to have, we can do much more than we often assume we can, mentally *and* physically. And that's true of seniors with low vision, too.

That's much different from the story people were telling each other twenty-five years ago. Twenty-five years ago, "disengagement theory" was popular. Disengagement theory held that as you became a senior, regardless of your own desires, you should reduce your activities, interests, and interactions with friends. The idea was that limiting yourself made accepting death easier. Not surprisingly, doctors have discovered that disengaging doesn't do much except make you miserable. In fact, they discovered not only that disengaging is bad for you but also that engaging is good for you. Pursuing the activities you enjoy, keeping and making new friends, and following a regular physical exercise routine can actually improve your memory and your mood, strengthen your balance and your stamina, boost your immune system, and increase your overall quality of life. And it doesn't matter if you're exercising in a wheelchair or if you start when you're ninety. You can still reap the benefits of engaging.

The Stories We Tell About Ourselves

Just as doctors and public policy makers tell stories about what it means to be older, we also tell stories about what it means to be ourselves. Sometimes we don't even realize we are telling stories. But whether we realize it or not, the stories we tell about ourselves are enormously influential, especially when we believe them. One of the most common stories people tell me about themselves is that they are less appealing and have less to offer others because they have low vision. "I don't go down to the dining room for lunch anymore because I'm afraid I'll spill coffee on myself," Rosa Garcia admitted quietly. "And besides, I can't see people too well, so I'm not sure I'll have much to say." After I talked with Rosa for a while, I discovered that she has opinions about the president and bilingual education and she loves the Chicago White Sox. She has a wonderfully warm smile and sixty years' experience as a mother, grandmother, and parish secretary. Why wouldn't anyone want to talk with her?

The Blindness Story

So where did Rosa get this idea that she's less appealing because she can't see as well as others do? She may have gotten it, along with her low vision, from macular degeneration. One of the challenges of AMD is that it comes with a whopper of a story: that macular degeneration causes blindness, that you can't really do anything if you're blind, and that you'll become an object of people's pity. This story isn't true, but it's so powerful that we often don't realize that we've adopted it.

My good friend Natalie Steele suddenly lost vision from macular degeneration last fall. The blow was so quick and sharp that she felt she would no longer be the same person to her friends if she made it plain to them. "I feel uncomfortable in restaurants," she admitted, "because I don't want to take out my lighted magnifier to read the menu. People will pity me, and I don't want their pity."

"They will see you the way you see yourself," I said. "If you pull out your magnifier with a flourish and say, 'Hey! Look at this! Isn't this the neatest tool? I just got it. It makes reading this menu so much easier,' they'll agree and they'll probably want one, too. After all, there are lots of restaurants dim enough that it's hard for anyone over fifty to see the menu."

People who know you care for you, not for what you can see. They are looking to you to tell them how to understand your vision loss. They want *your* story, not some generic story of blindness or some story that's foisted on you. As for strangers, they usually aren't looking. If you do run into people who dish out pity or seem uncomfortable with your vision, you can pity them right back, because if they live long enough, someday they will experience a disability, too. And that day will be doubly hard for them.

A month ago, Natalie took her magnifier out at a luncheon with friends. The waiter graciously appeared at her side with a beautifully designed large-print menu and quietly slipped it to her. She felt as if she might start crying from elation and relief. He had treated her with immediate respect, without a drop of patronizing pity. I shouted, "Hallelujah!" It's about time restaurants realized that their patrons need large-print menus. Isn't this the way it should always be?

The Macular Degeneration Slide

If you adopt the ready-made macular degeneration story that this condition means you can't really do anything, then you're at risk for what I call the macular degeneration slide. The beginning of the slide looks like commonsense adjusting, but it skids pretty quickly into something much more insidious and self-limiting.

John Patrick Reynolds, who goes by Pat, came to our low-vision rehabilitation program this year with his daughter, Sheila. "He talks about how distraught he is not to renew his driver's license," Sheila told me in the hallway, "but it's giving up hunting that's killing him."

"I have to give it up, like the driving," Pat told me when I asked him about it, "I can't shoot anything. I can't see the damn target."

"So what do you like most about hunting?" I asked.

Pat talked about how much he loves being outdoors with his buddies. How they've gone up north for a week together each season for twenty-eight years. Barbecuing in the crisp night air, hiking every day, crouching in the leaves. He loves the quiet, the smell of the woods, the company of good friends.

"How many deer did you all shoot last season?" I asked.

"Oh, we only got two. There's five of us, but three guys didn't get anything."

"So," I said, "you have low vision. What's their excuse?"

Pat started to chuckle.

"Seriously," I said, "if you all have been hiking through the woods together for twenty-eight years and you can still hike . . . why not go? Looks like you won't be the only one who doesn't hit anything. If accurate shooting was really a prerequisite for this trip, there'd only be two people on it."

Don't get on macular degeneration slide. Don't give up the things that are important to you just because you think you should or because you think you need to—explore your options first. Don't cancel your newspaper subscription before you find out if you can read it with a CCTV. Don't give up reading *Reader's Digest* before you try their big-print edition. Don't give up a trip with your buddies before you realize that you can still go and have a great time anyway.

The Power of Positive Stories

Inspirational speakers like Norman Vincent Peale and Dale Carnegie and religious leaders like Billy Graham have been telling us for decades that positive thinking is powerful. That's why every major religious tradition teaches love and forgiveness, because these are the two most powerful stories of living: that we love and are loved and that we forgive the failings in ourselves and others. Listen to the positive stories you hear about seniors in the world and tell positive stories about yourself and about what you can do. We're all human; we all have doubts, insecurities, and embarrassments. We always will. But don't make them the only truth in your life.

When Stories Come to Life

The inspiring guide *Secrets of Becoming a Late Bloomer* encourages all seniors to be as active as they want to be, doing the things they want to do. The book tells the story of Jack, who has macular degeneration and becomes a reading tutor for children. Jack's the third person I've found with low vision from AMD who tutors reading. It's a brilliant idea, actually. In Jack's case, he decided that he'd always liked children, so he contacted a volunteer placement service. They sent him to meet with the local elementary school principal. The principal told Jack that what the school really needed was reading tutors, but she assumed that Jack's low vision meant he couldn't help. "I suppose the idea's completely out of the question," she concluded. But Jack explained that the children could read to him aloud and he would correct their pronunciation. If a child couldn't read a word, Jack would ask him or her to spell it aloud and would help the child figure out the word. This tutoring strategy works well for Jack and his students, and it works well for other people with low vision who also tutor reading. When I read Jack's story, I realized I was reading a story about how one man managed to tell a different story about his potential than the one someone else assumed was true. And I realized that Jack's story illustrates visual rehabilitation at its best.

Visual Rehabilitation

As you'll discover when you turn to part III of this book, visual rehabilitation is about learning new skills, like reading with low vision, and using new products, like magnifiers, indoor floodlight bulbs, and CCTVs. Those are the nuts and bolts. At its heart, though, visual rehabilitation is really about saying, Hey, world, this is what I need and this is what I'd like to do, and then not taking *no* for an answer, at least not easily. It's about telling your own story of what you can do, rather than listening to someone else's.

As you already know, telling your own story isn't always easy. Macular degeneration can turn the world upside down, making the familiar seem unfamiliar and the safe feel precarious. It can make you much more aware of what you can't do than what you can do. Macular degeneration can make living in your own community seem like traveling in a foreign country without the glamour of flying somewhere. If you're in Greece, ordering dinner at a restaurant when you can't read the local language is exotic and exciting, but it loses its appeal if it happens in your hometown. Visual rehabilitation is about putting more things in the "can do" column than the "can't do" one and developing the tools to tell your own story. After all, Jack makes volunteer tutoring look simple, but he had to get to the elementary school somehow and he had to have a bit of confidence to stand up and explain how he was going to tutor reading without having his central vision. Where did those skills come from? They came from visual rehabilitation.

Telling Your Own Story

The story you tell about yourself or what you'd like to do doesn't have to be the same as Jack's. Not everyone wants to be a reading tutor or a volunteer in any capacity (although the rewards can be invaluable). When I asked Rosa Garcia what she would like to do, she said she'd like to make dinner for her family. My father likes to bowl. Grace Olsen likes to play bridge with a few friends using big-print cards. Sam and Rachel Weinberg like to go to the opera; they also enjoy traveling to Elder Hostel courses. Zelda Grant likes to raise Cain in her yoga class, her support group, and her book club (she listens to the books on tape, while the other members read regular paperbacks). Your own story can be whatever you want it to be, but make it about living fully in whatever ways you would most enjoy.

TAKING RISKS

We tend to recognize physical risks—like walking on icy sidewalks—as risks, but we don't often talk about social risks as risks. Those slide under the table. But social risks are a big concern for many people with macular degeneration. No one avoids them. My father has asked a mannequin for directions to the men's department, taken the wrong bus, taken a sip of someone else's drink, hugged a stranger, passed by old pals on the street, and missed bowling pins. But none of these mistakes have cost him friends or dignity. The answer to almost any social situation is to be straightforward about your vision and remember that fears are *fears*, not reflections of what will really happen or what others will really think.

Keep Your Sense of Humor

If you can see the risks of low vision with a light-hearted eye, at least sometimes, they become much less pressing. Francie Klein, who is a marvelous cook, once made cherry pie for a party with kidney beans instead of cherries. "I had a good laugh about it," she said. "I'm lucky because my father taught me how to live with macular degeneration. He had it, too. He once took a bite out of a cork coaster, mistaking it for an almond cookie. "Dad!" I said, "That's a coaster!" "Well, thank goodness," he said, "I thought your cooking was going to pot."

Let Others Know You Have Low Vision

If you have macular degeneration, no one else can tell. People will assume you can see them and you may pass old friends on the street. Tell everyone you know that you have low vision and you may not recognize them. They have to say hello directly and introduce themselves. After a while, your friends and acquaintances will adjust. Newcomers may be temporarily confused, so you may always run into this problem. But any person who gets upset because you didn't say hello first or respond when they waved need to have their head examined. You can tell them I said so. Besides, they'll feel foolish if they get macular degeneration and need your advice. You may think I'm kidding, but I'm not. Whatever you do, though, don't squash your own personality with worry. Go get 'em.

Don't Hesitate to Ask for Assistance

Do everything you can for yourself, and don't hesitate to ask for assistance. That sounds like contradictory advice, but it's really not. Sometimes you need a bit of assistance to do something for yourself. Better to ask a store clerk to read a price tag than to avoid shopping altogether. Better to ask a pedestrian which bus is pulling up than to avoid public transportation. Better to ask a family member or friend if your lipstick is on right than to avoid going outside.

This last example touches a nerve for many people. If you've taken pride in your appearance all your life, as most of us have, you may feel chagrined to find out that you're wearing brown socks with a blue suit or wearing a sweater that needs a trip to the cleaner's. But let's be honest. It's not a character weakness to mismatch colors or have a piece of string or a spot on your clothes. Other people are unlikely to even notice; and if they do, they are unlikely to think anything of it at all. We always care more about our own appearances than anyone else does.

If you are very concerned, ask others to tell you if they notice anything amiss in your appearance. Remember, it's no different from fully sighted people having a smudge of chocolate on their face or a mark on the back of their skirt. They rely on someone else to tell them, so ask them to tell you. Make a deal with your family, friends, and neighbors that you want them to tell you if they notice anything amiss in your appearance because it helps you to know. I made this deal with my father and we're both so used to it now that we don't think twice. He feels more comfortable knowing I'll tell him, and I feel more comfortable knowing I can tell him.

Be Honest with Friends and Family

Dostoevsky once wrote that "much unhappiness has come into the world because of bewilderment and things left unsaid." I often talk with people who are reluctant to tell their friends and family much about their low vision for fear of distressing or burdening them. Sometimes they aren't being honest about small things. But sometimes those small things pile up and become big things.

When Grace first lost her driver's license from low vision, she decided not to attend bridge club anymore because she couldn't drive herself. Since she would never know whether or not she would be a burden, Grace declined her friend Lily's offer of a ride. Besides, Grace reasoned, she couldn't see regular playing cards anyway and she didn't want to ask the group to play with big-print cards. For several weeks, Lily called her, but Grace held firm. Grace's stoic determination to remain independent was admirable but misguided. She managed to make herself very lonely, and Lily, too.

I happen to know Lily and know that she really enjoyed Grace's company and enjoyed having dinner with Grace after bridge club. "Grace won't come to bridge club anymore," Lily told me when I saw her outside the grocery store. "I guess her vision is going and she doesn't feel like playing cards. I tried to call her, but she won't come." There was something resigned and sad in Lily's voice. As she turned and walked away, I watched her tiny sloping shoulders disappear down the street. Lily cares a lot more about Grace's company, I thought, than she does about whether or not Grace can drive herself to bridge club, and Grace isn't listening.

Fortunately, Grace finally realized that she has more to offer her friends than perfect vision. Today Grace takes a cab to bridge club, the group plays with big-print cards, and Lily drives her home after they've had dinner together. And they are both happier. There is nothing independent about forcing yourself to stay home in order to avoid being dependent. Don't shut out your friends. Instead, tell them what you need and look for alternative ways to do what you want to do.

CHOOSING TO LIVE

Choosing to live doesn't mean never being angry, frustrated, or upset. But it does mean recognizing your responses and realizing that you have choices. You can't choose your vision, but you still have choices. In fact, low vision asks us to do one thing above all: it asks us to make a single big choice that ultimately determines all of our other choices, our lives, and the lives of those closest to us.

Tom Perski, M.A., the founder of Macular Degeneration International in Tucson, told me about a couple who came in to his program for counseling.

"The wife was saying that she was so tired of driving all the time since her husband gave it up from macular degeneration. But it wasn't the road that was tiring her out; it was him. He was constantly yelling at her while she was trying to drive, *'Turn here!'* or *'Slow down!'* or *'What the heck are you doing?'*

"So I told the couple a story about a gal I was dating shortly after I lost my own license in my twenties from the juvenile form of macular degeneration. We were driving somewhere and I was yelling at this gal just the same way. She finally pulled over and told me to get out of the car. I did, and she drove off. She left me there on the side of the road for an hour.

"After that gal drove off, I sat on the side of that road all burned up. But that hour changed my whole life. I realized that I had to take responsibility for my own anger and frustration and stop venting it on the people closest to me. I realized that I was free to either live or to drain the life from those around me, and I chose to live."

Tom's experience rings true for everyone with macular degeneration and for many other people as well. We will all someday sit on the side of the road with a choice. We can either choose to let vision loss or another life-changing collision darken everything we feel and do for years to come or we can choose to live. Really live. We can choose to let light and life and laughter and love in again.

Lose the Rigidity

Macular degeneration is not what anybody ordered for retirement. Nobody sits back after forty years of work and says, "Hmm. What I really need now is a colossal life challenge. I'd really like some of that low vision." So when it hits, it can have a chilling effect, like a winter whiteout, especially on a marriage. It can freeze a couple rigidly into place.

I have seen husbands with macular degeneration frozen to their recliners, refusing to go anywhere, refusing to dance or walk in the park. I've seen wives with macular degeneration frozen in their kitchens, believing that if they can't make exactly the same dishes exactly the same way then nothing is good anymore. I've seen husbands with full vision frozen with assumptions about what their wives can and can't see. "She's just not trying. She can see that," they'll say. And I've

seen wives with full vision frozen rigid with unforgiving anger, reducing their husbands to tears
for trivial mistakes, for not seeing unwashed
spots on the dishes or failing to fix a doorknob
correctly.

You've got to lose the rigidity. It's the first
thing that goes when you choose to live. There is
no longer one right way to do things. There is no
longer one right role. Like Inez Toscano, who
learned to drive for the first time at seventy-five
after her husband, Joe, got macular degeneration,
you might need to take on new tasks. Or like Bixley Bennett, who revised her recipe collection to
feature the dishes that are easiest for her to make
with low vision, you might need to start doing the
same tasks differently.

Most of all, you've got to communicate. Without communicating, it's difficult to do anything
but stand frozen in place. Communicating isn't
easy; sometimes it takes counseling with a therapist or clergy member. We may never see things
the same way—but with compassion for our
selves and each other we can still love and maybe
even laugh together. And isn't that the essence of
living?

I am reminded of Sam and Rachel Weinberg
when they came in one day.

Sam very earnestly told me, "We've always
been very independent of one another, but now we
often work as a team."

Rachel winked and squeezed Sam's hand affectionately. "Yes, it's teamwork," she said, "but it's also 'Rachel! Rachel! Could you double-check these figures please? Rachel! Rachel! Could you come and look at this please? Rachel! Rachel!' I might change my name to Veronica."

Losing the rigidity doesn't mean losing yourself. It's not about faking your feelings or becoming Mother Teresa. It's about choosing to live. Macular degeneration may choose our vision for us, but in the end we choose what we see with it. The more flexible we are, the more we will see.

Live Through Exercise

If you are older and have low vision, you may assume that you can't exercise or that it wouldn't be safe. Not true! Actually, exercise is really important for people with macular degeneration, because low vision often reduces your activity and mobility. If you don't make an effort, you may become more sedentary, and that's not good for your overall health. Exercise improves your stamina and balance, it helps stabilize sleep patterns and insulin levels, it improves your outlook and mood, and it increases the length and improves the quality of your life. Not only that, but you don't have to be an athlete to reap the benefits of exercise. You just have to start exercising. The hardest part of exercising, however, is starting. The next hardest part is sticking with it for at least one month. After a month, your body will become more accustomed to exercising and you will feel better on a daily basis. Stay with a program for at least six months to a year. If you stop, you can begin again and still benefit. Your body is remarkably elastic; you just have to give it a chance. You will see changes.

Always check with your doctor before you begin an exercise program. Begin modestly, and increase your program gradually. If you are not accustomed to exercising, begin with five minutes of walking or riding an Exercycle four to five days a week. When this becomes easy, increase your time gradually until you reach twenty to thirty minutes four to five days a week. Talk to your doctor about adding gentle stretches to your program to loosen the muscles that you use and prevent injury or consider enrolling in a gentle stretching class. If you cannot walk or are worried about falling, consider lifting leg or arm weights. You can buy lightweight ones with Velcro straps for your ankles and wrists, or you can hold light arm weights. You may also want to try a stationary bike, pool aerobics class, swimming, or pool jogging (see chapter 14 for details).

Live Through Love

Whenever I think my sexiest days are over, I think of Georgette. She came in for a visual rehabilitation appointment the day after her seventy-fifth birthday with a rock the size of Texas on her ring finger.

"Congratulations!" I said warmly, "You're getting married!"

She looked at me with some horror. "Oh, no, my dear. I'm engaged. But I am absolutely *not* getting married. I washed and cooked and cleaned for my husband for forty-seven years, God rest his soul, and that was enough work for me."

"But you're engaged."

"Yes, of course I'm engaged!" Georgette said with enthusiasm. "It's wonderful to be engaged. We have so much fun together. We go to dinner all the time and we just love to travel. He treats me just like a princess."

"A princess?"

"At first he didn't want to go out, you know, because his vision is no good, either. He can't drive anymore. So he didn't want to go out. But I'll tell you, I was thinking, Honey, it's not the car that makes the man. Oh, no. And you know the best part? He thinks I'm beautiful, so it's just as well that he doesn't see every wrinkle. He thinks I'm as beautiful as I was twenty years ago, and sometimes when I'm with him, I even think so, too. Of course, he looks pretty good to me, too, you know, and that's not so bad."

Georgette winked at me. And then she smiled this wonderful smile and her eyes just twinkled.

Until then, I hadn't realized that some things

might actually be *better* with low vision, and Georgette had clearly found one of them.

Live Through Reaching Out

Sometimes the best defense is a good offense. Zelda Grant knew this when she started marching around the world asking what was available for her now that she has low vision. But you don't need to be Zelda to enjoy the benefits of a good offense. You just have to be you, really you. Dolores Lopez loves going to her church services, but she couldn't see who was there anymore, which made her uncomfortable. So she hit upon a brilliant offensive strategy: she volunteers as a greeter for the services she attends, so everyone comes up to her and introduces themselves on their way in the door and now she knows who's there and everyone knows her.

Bixley Bennett was feeling frustrated because she wasn't seeing her friends quite as often as she used to when she could drive. So she hit upon a brilliant offensive strategy: she began volunteering through her local senior center calling folks who are homebound. "I thought I would do it as a community service to keep busy, and I feel less sorry for myself by talking to people in worse straits than I am," Bixley confessed. "But it's changed my life. I've made new friends. I love talking with them every week. I call them my angels."

When you choose to live, choose to reach out. Look for opportunities, not for limitations. Choose a good offense.

Live Through Faith

When I first met Evangeline, who has low vision from macular degeneration, she told me a ribald joke. At ninety, she didn't miss a beat. After an hour, she announced that she couldn't stay any longer because she'd miss her luncheon date with her gentleman friend. "Have you any advice for the younger generation?" I asked, figuring that I could take the advice myself and be as vibrant in twenty-five years as she is today. She smiled and paused, clearly choosing her words.

"Yes," she finally said, "I will tell you what I tell my great-grandchildren. Pray to the Holy Family."

"That's it?" I said.

"Yes, that's it," she said. And out she went.

The Holy Family? Not being Catholic, I didn't see an immediate use for the advice. But as I met more and more people with low vision, I remembered Evangeline's words. I began to understand that faith plays an important part in how we experience life and how we experience low vision. By faith I mean the belief that you are valuable as an *individual no matter what* and that your life has meaning. Faith protects us from unnecessary anxiety. Faith forgives us and makes sense of fate. Faith is also a muscle that we can exercise: it can grow strong through time and through engagement with the activities and people you enjoy.

Whatever faith you profess, I tell my patients, I have faith in you. You are our role models. We look to you, as I looked to Evangeline, to see how to handle being older and losing vision. You are the first generation to do so. And we're right behind you.

CHAPTER 7

Sixteen Tips for Family and Friends

A faithful friend is the medicine of life.
—Ecclesiasticus 6:16

Many family members and friends of people with AMD have asked me what they can do to help. Here are sixteen tips:

1. Be Direct About Vision

Ask your friend or family member what they can and can't see so that you know. Don't worry about using phrases that emphasize vision, like "Did you see Zelda yesterday?"

2. Identify Yourself and Say Hello

Take the initiative to say hello and identify yourself when you see your family member or friend. And don't always assume that other seniors can see you. At the very least, one out of every twelve seniors over seventy-five has low vision.

3. Say Everything You Want to Convey

Give clear verbal directions and avoid vague

replies like "It's over there." Don't assume that your friend or family member can read your facial expressions or gestures. Express your reactions aloud. Say everything that you want the other person to know.

4. Use Black Felt-Tip or Ink Pens and Print in Clear Lettering

Always write notes or letters to your family member or friend in black-felt tip or ink pen or black computer print. Print clearly in letters large enough for your friend or family member to see. Don't use colored paper or pens, ballpoint pens, or pencils, since they are very difficult to see. For birthdays and holidays, consider calling instead of sending a card.

5. Give Low-Vision Gifts

Consider giving low-vision gifts such as talking calculators, watches, clocks, thermometers, weight scales, and computer software. You could also give large-button or automatic dialing phones or large-print cards, clocks, calendars, or address books. There are all kinds of other gifts to choose from in the low-vision catalogs listed in appendix C. Alternatively, consider giving a book on tape or tickets to a concert or helping purchase a CCTV.

6. Keep the Environment Predictable

A predictable environment makes a big difference for anyone with low vision. Many people can compensate for less vision by relying on their knowledge of the environment. Help your friend or family member keep his or her home (and yours if you live together) as predictable as possible. Keep frequently used items like house keys, salt shakers, and trash bags in designated places. Put things away after you use them, and close cupboard and stairwell doors. If you are a guest, return any item you move to the place you found it, even a coffee table book that looks merely decorative. If the color of the book contrasts with the coffee table, your friend or family member may be using it to see the coffee table more clearly.

7. Offer Your Arm; Don't Take Theirs

When you walk with your friend or family member, offer your arm. Don't take his or her arm because you may throw them off balance. This guideline for walking applies to all of low-vision life: offer help where it's necessary, but don't just do it yourself.

8. Don't Just Do for Your Parent

Enable your parent to do as much for him or herself as possible. Don't assume that because of low vision your parent isn't capable, and don't foster that assumption in your parent. If your parent wants to take out the trash, walk to the cleaner's, mow the lawn, cook a family dinner, volunteer at a local center, or run a manufacturing company, so much the better! As busy adult children, we often feel like less responsibility would be a relief for us, so that must be true for our parents. But having nothing to work toward can be deathly boring. Too much responsibility is stressful, but too little is unhealthy. Don't take away anyone's reason for having to be up and about in the morning. And don't take away anyone's ability to help you. Take the time you would have spent doing your parent's chores and share some activity you both enjoy.

9. Share Activities You Both Enjoy

Find new or old activities that please both of you. Call your friend or family member and make a date. Here are a few suggestions:

- Dine out.

- Attend a wine tasting or food fair.

- Go to the symphony, the opera, or a jazz concert.

- Visit a botanical garden or garden together in the yard.

- Golf, bowl; swim; lift weights; walk in the park.

- Listen to a book on tape or a radio show together.

- Do a crossword puzzle together.

- Play cards, chess, checkers, or large-print Scrabble.

- Demonstrate at a political rally.

- Get facials and manicures.

- Go to a lecture series, a book reading, or a poetry reading.

- Go to a baseball or football game (you can also listen to commentary on the radio either at home or in the stadium).

- Take yoga, stretching classes, tai chi, water aerobics, or meditation classes.

- Start or join a salon, discussion group, or support group.

- Attend religious services.

- Volunteer at a local charity.

- Sail or skydive, with a qualified instructor, of course.

10. Encourage Interests

When you lose vision, you don't lose your physical or mental energy. Encourage your friend or family member to maintain old interests and cultivate new ones. Encourage hobbies, volunteer work, membership in senior clubs or support groups, and reading and listening to broadcasts, books, newspaper articles, and magazines (see appendix B for the many options and services available). We so often think of paid jobs or parenting as significant and hobbies or interests as optional, but they're not. Everybody needs to be a part of their community, be aware of it, and be alive in it. When you're younger, jobs and parenting may take up most of your time, but when you're a senior you have time for other interests. And whatever you spend your time doing is just as important for the quality of your life today as your job was for the quality of your life in earlier years. For adult children especially, retirement may look like heaven and having no role may seem like sweet relief. But just being retired without any interests or just living comfortably in a tidy apartment, without much stimulation, or just coping with low vision as a full-time preoccupation is a short-term recipe for boredom and a long-term recipe for personal distress and crisis. Being alive is the sum total of our actions, mental and physical, in this world. Be active; encourage action.

11. Realize the Importance of Friends

If you are a friend, realize how important you are. If you are an adult child, realize that everyone needs friends. We are so used to thinking of family as our fortress and friends as nice but not as necessary that we may discount their importance. While family is often our fortress, friends may be equally so and sometimes even more important for seniors' happiness and longevity. I often meet seniors who have moved out of their communities and into apartments in their adult children's neighborhoods. The move initially solves a number of problems: the adult child feels more confident caring for his or her parent, the parent feels safer, and keeping accurate banking records and troubleshooting with doctors may be easier. But over time, as the adult child returns to his or her responsibilities, working full-time or shuttling children to school, the senior parent spends the vast majority of the day alone.

Without any friends, seniors are prone to loneliness *regardless of how much their adult children try to meet their needs*. And loneliness is not a good thing. It does not make you very excited about living and may even lead to clinical depression. Keeping old friends and making new ones should be at the very top of the priority list when considering living arrangements. I strongly recommend that seniors stay connected to their local communities, move to senior residences that feature plenty of social events and encourage meeting people, or actively work to make new friends, join new groups, and engage in new activities with others wherever they move. Adult children would do their parents a greater service helping them make or keep friends than almost anything else.

12. Watch for Depression

Depression is very common among people with macular degeneration. Many people experience a short period of depression as they adjust to vision loss, but many others experience prolonged periods of depression. Be aware of changes in your friend's or family member's emotional state, sleeping patterns, weight, or behavior. Excessive worry, bouts of crying, listlessness or disinterest, low motivation, pessimism or snippiness, social withdrawal, a refusal to communicate or an excessively stiff upper lip, moping, and helplessness all may signal depression. Depression is not healthy for anyone. See chapter 6 and talk directly to your friend or family member about your concerns. If your spouse or parent appears depressed, make an appointment with his or her doctor, pursue visual rehabilitation, and get your loved one out into the world or involved in new activities (even if you have to give a gentle push).

13. Take Care of Yourself, Too

If you are married to or living with someone who has vision loss, you may be at risk for depression, too. So be your own best friend, too, and look out for your well-being by following the same steps you would for your loved one. Even if you're fine, you may feel like your life has turned upside down sometimes or you're faced with challenges you hadn't expected and you need some support.

That's why visual rehabilitation should be for families, too. See if your local program has a family support group or consider starting your own using the guidelines in chapter 6. You may also want to join one of the macular degeneration organizations listed in appendix A or the on-line community MD People. The more active you are with your spouse, partner, or roommate in visual rehabilitation, the better both your lives will be.

14. Participate in Visual Rehabilitation

Participating in visual rehabilitation in the broadest sense means fostering a sense of independence, self-determination, and joy. That does not mean that people who are successfully pursuing visual rehabilitation need to prove that they can do it all by themselves, live on their own, or get a volunteer job. But it does mean living as fully as possible. There are many practical things you can do to be a part of your family member or friend's visual rehabilitation. Here are just a few suggestions:

- Read a chapter from part III of this book together and work as a team to implement the suggestions. This may include rearranging the furniture, closets, or clothing, taping down area rugs, installing new lighting fixtures, choosing contrasting tablecloths or dishes, or labeling dials, bottles, electronics, and appliances.

- Encourage your friend or family member to continue reading by completing the Reading Workshop in chapter 10 together. Help set up a well-lit reading space and facilitate trying new visual aids like a CCTV. Encourage participation in the NLS or CNIB library program (see appendix B).

- If you have a computer, consider reprinting your friend or family member's recipes or addresses in large type and collecting them in a binder or having them bound at a copy shop. Alternatively, help set up a computer workstation with Internet access and low-vision software (see appendix C).

- Encourage your friend or family member to exercise regularly.

- Help your friend or family member learn to use public transportation.

- If you live together, tell your friend or family member what he or she can do to help you with chores or other responsibilities.

- Talk directly to your friend or family member about his or her experiences and feelings about low vision. Talk about your feelings, too.

15. Help Start a Support Group

Support groups are a fantastic way to build community. At a low-vision support group, your friend or family member would have the chance to talk to people who have walked a mile in his or her shoes and can understand the experience. Support groups are great places to vent, to laugh, to get new solutions for daily challenges and new ideas for living. They are also important sources of support for spouses or roommates of people with vision loss. It's very comforting to talk to the natives, as author Bernie Siegel calls anyone who shares a common experience with you. Contact your local visual rehabilitation program to ask about support groups or join the Internet community MD People (see appendix A). If there is no support group in your area, that doesn't mean there aren't any other people with low vision there. It just means that no one is getting the benefit of a support group. Why not help start one? See chapter 6 for guidelines.

16. Keep Your Sense of Humor

We are all prone to taking life too seriously. Very few people get to the end of their lives wishing they had been more earnest, more worried, or more self-conscious. We all try so hard to get it right the first time, to avoid misfortune and mistakes, to look good in public. Sometimes we forget to laugh. Laugh from your belly, and let your friend or family member see the daily humor in this busy, unpredictable, ridiculous, profound, heartbreaking, and heartwarming experience we call living.

CHAPTER 8

I See Purple Flowers Everywhere: The Many Visions of Charles Bonnet Syndrome

"Do you ever see anything you know is not there but looks real anyway?" I asked Sam Weinberg when he came to the Low Vision Living Program.

"No," he said, looking at his wife, Rachel, and fidgeting with his sweater.

"Oh," I said casually, "I just asked because many people with macular degeneration see things they know are not there. I call it phantom vision, but the technical term is *Charles Bonnet Syndrome.*"

"Is this syndrome an early sign of Alzheimer's?" Sam asked pointedly, still looking at Rachel. Rachel began to look at the clock on the wall. They had been in our office for nearly two hours and Rachel felt it was already past lunchtime. She picked up her coat.

"Absolutely not," I said firmly. "Charles Bonnet Syndrome has nothing to do with mental agility or stability. When you have phantom vision, your mind is fine; it's your eyes that are playing tricks on you. It's a side effect of low vision."

"Well," Sam admitted quickly, "I see little monkeys with red hats and blue coats playing in the front yard. I've seen them for eighteen months."

"*What!*" Rachel's eyes about popped out of her head, and she dropped her coat. "*Little monkeys in the front yard?*"

"Well . . . um," Sam continued, "sometimes I see them in the living room, too."

What Is Charles Bonnet Syndrome?

Charles Bonnet was an eighteenth-century Swiss naturalist and philosopher whose grandfather, Charles Lullin, had low vision from cataracts. In 1769, Bonnet described his grandfather's curious experience of seeing men, women, birds, and buildings that he knew were not there. Later in his life, Bonnet's own vision also deteriorated and he experienced phantom visions similar to his grandfather's. How could this happen? Curiously, Charles Bonnet's discovery didn't capture medical attention at the time. But 150 years later, in the 1930s, his files were dusted off, and he was credited with being the first person to describe the syndrome that came to be named for him. The medical origins of Charles Bonnet Syndrome, however, remained unclear.

Today there are several suggested causes. The most convincing holds that the syndrome is analogous to phantom limb phenomena. People who have a limb amputated may still feel their toes or fingers or itching on an arm that no longer exists. This happens because the limb's nerves are still active, spontaneously firing signals to the brain, which the brain dutifully interprets. So, too, with the eyes. When retinal cells become impaired, and are no longer able to receive and relay visual images to the brain or when any other element of the visual system ceases to function optimally, the system begins firing off images on its own.

The funny thing about these images is that they are often not related to a person's life at all. Sam's monkeys, for example, were entirely original creations. He couldn't remember ever seeing these monkeys before, and he wasn't a particular fan of monkeys anyway. He found them surprising at first, especially since they seemed so vivid and lifelike, but after a while they became amusing. Since they were so clearly not real monkeys, Sam wasn't too worried about his own mind, but he was afraid that others would be, especially Rachel.

How Common Is Charles Bonnet Syndrome?

This syndrome is very common. Studies place the number somewhere between 10 percent and

40 percent of people with low vision. Twenty percent of my low-vision patients have Charles Bonnet Syndrome. My research suggests that it is more likely to appear if you have a visual acuity between 20/120 and 20/400 (see chapter 1 for an explanation of the 20/20 visual acuity measurement scale). This may be because eyes with a visual acuity between these two measurements still have a great deal of power but aren't receiving or relaying as many images from the world as they used to. As a result, they may be adding some images of their own. We have no reliable way to know ahead of time whether you will see images, how frequently these images will occur, or how long they will last. You may never experience Charles Bonnet Syndrome, you may have it for only a few months, or you may have it for years. You may see images only a few times a month or a few times a week for a few minutes, or you may see images every day.

Are You Sure This Has Nothing to Do with Psychiatry?

Yes, phantom vision, or Charles Bonnet Syndrome, is properly a side effect of vision loss only. Unfortunately, since ophthalmologists have rarely investigated this syndrome in the twentieth century, some psychiatric studies have used the term to describe people with visual hallucinations, people with normal vision who see things they believe are actually real. To set the record straight, I'd like to return to the six criteria for Charles Bonnet Syndrome outlined by Naville in 1873. You can use them to determine whether or not you are experiencing phantom vision. Do the images that appear to you have the following six characteristics?

1. They occur when you are fully conscious and wide awake, often during broad daylight.

2. They do not deceive you; you are aware that they are not real.

3. They occur in combination with normal perception. For example, you may see a sidewalk clearly but find it covered with dots, flowers, or faces.

4. They are exclusively visual and do not appear in combination with any sounds or bizarre sensations.

5. They appear and disappear without obvious cause.

6. They are amusing or annoying but not grotesque.

Since ophthalmology has paid so little attention to Charles Bonnet Syndrome, many doctors don't realize how common it really is and some may not be familiar with it at all. When I gave a poster presentation of the drawings in this chapter at the American Academy of Ophthalmology's Annual Meeting in the fall of 1997, several ophthalmologists stopped to express their surprise at hearing about phantom vision for the first time.

What Do People with Charles Bonnet Syndrome See?

A 1994 Dutch study of Charles Bonnet Syndrome listed the following images seen by participants: miniature chimney sweeps, farmers, strolling children, teddy bears, windmills, chairs, women in woolly hats, and men in striped pajamas. My patients at Low Vision Living have reported seeing cartoon characters, flowers in the bathroom sink, hands rubbing each other, waterfalls and mountains, tigers, maple trees in vibrant autumn foliage, yellow polka dots, row houses, a dinner party, and brightly colored balloons. Many people see faces or life-size figures that they've never seen before. One of the most remarkable qualities of these figures is that they almost always wear pleasant expressions and often make eye contact with the viewer. Menacing behavior, grotesque shapes, and scenes of violent conflict are not, to my knowledge, a part of this syndrome.

Usually the same image or set of images reappears to each person, sometimes in the same places or at the same time of day. Sam's monkeys usually materialized around sunset, cavorting across the lawn or around the big blue easy chair by the fireplace. They stayed for ten or twenty minutes several times a week for two years and then began to appear less frequently. Sometimes the images change or multiple images appear. While Sam saw only monkeys, Joe Toscano saw chestnut horses and small rabbits on the kitchen walls. They were soon replaced by willow trees at a riverbank. Sometimes the images are exactly to scale and sometimes larger or smaller than life. Sometimes the images become smaller the farther away they appear, and sometimes they become larger. Joe's horses looked like children's toys at a distance of ten feet, but as they galloped outside they became Clydesdales and then stallions worthy of Gulliver.

Treating Charles Bonnet Syndrome

Fortunately, most people find Charles Bonnet Syndrome largely untroubling. Since the images it produces are usually pretty or lighthearted, many actually find them amusing or enjoyable. If, however, you find yourself frustrated or anxious, do not hesitate to discuss phantom vision with your doctor. Although no drug treatment has been demonstrated to work for everyone, the best option appears to be low-dose Haldol. Usually explanation and reassurance are sufficient.

Sometimes Charles Bonnet Syndrome images can become confused with dream images. For example, several of my patients have reported frightening moments when they thought they saw a man standing in their bedroom or hallway. These men, however, were often dark-clad or indistinct figures that appeared as the patient was relaxing on a couch, dozing, or in bed waiting to fall asleep or just awaking. These figures were probably residual dream images that reflected very normal fears of crime or loneliness. They are not, however, typical of Charles Bonnet Syndrome. As Zelda Grant put it, "Shadowy men in my bedroom? Don't be ridiculous! I see fully dressed Canadian Mounties in my bedroom with long gold sabers, big gold buttons, and stiff-brimmed blue hats. They have nice wide shoulders. They're a good-looking group."

A CHARLES BONNET PORTRAIT GALLERY

When Grace Olsen came to Low Vision Living, I asked her the same question I asked Sam Weinberg: "Do you ever see anything you know is not there but looks real anyway?"

She eyed me dryly. "Yes," she said, with an air of great patience, "but my problem is that I can't see things that *are* there. I do not much care if the kitchen sink is full of American flags. I would like to know how I can see my granddaughter's photo."

Touché! Grace was right, of course, but she

was also surprised and comforted to hear that other people with low vision saw things in their sinks, too. Like Sam and Rachel Weinberg, Grace had never heard of Charles Bonnet Syndrome before; she supposed she might be the only one, so she had never shared the images she saw.

After I opened a set of felt-tip markers, we spent some time together talking about low vision and about the extraordinary set of flags, plaids, and bars of music Grace saw everywhere. The vivid colors Grace used to draw her patterns helped me understand her experience in greater detail. As she drew, Grace talked about her years as a young documentary artist for the Works Progress Administration during the Depression and her love of all things blue: irises, jays, and oceans. Her words made me wonder anew at what a strange and stunning gift sight really is: what things we have seen, what things we remember, and what things we never expected to see. Since Grace left her drawings with me, I've asked other people with macular degeneration to depict the images they see and to talk about their experience with Charles Bonnet Syndrome. I'd like to share their drawings and words with you.

Grace Olsen's Turquoise Squares and Bars of Music

I was in the hospital a few years ago for pneumonia. I remember sitting in my bed, waiting for lunch, when I saw light turquoise and lime green squares on the ceiling. *That's strange,* I thought, but I wasn't feeling well, so I just closed my eyes. A few weeks later, I was mixing salad dressing in the kitchen and the same checkered pattern reappeared on the floor. Now I see it everywhere. Sometimes it's quite small, a few inches at most, and sometimes it covers a whole bedspread. I can't remember ever seeing these squares in my life. I thought they might be from one of my drawings or photographs, but I never drew abstract patterns, and my photographs were always black-and-white. Then I thought they came from a quilt. I used to quilt with a group, and often toured antique shops. But the lime green in this check is too rich, too goldish- or brownish-tinted, more like an abstract painting than a color of thread. After I became quite used

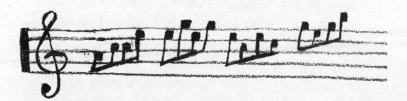

Grace Olsen's bars of music.

to the checks, I began to see an ornate
bar of music. *Good grief!* That's all I could
think. I spent my childhood praying that
my mother would let me give up the
piano. I hated practicing so much. Why in
the world would I see a bar of music? I
have tried to read the music I see, but it
doesn't seem to play a particular tune.
Just shapes, decorative shapes.

Zelda Grant's Redbrick Building

When I was a child in North Carolina
during the Depression, I had a very old
maiden aunt, Isabel. I thought she didn't
have much fun, because she never ate
cake when she came to our house. She
lived in a redbrick home for the elderly. I
believed that if you didn't have any
money they sent you there. I remember
my parents whispering to one another
about money and debts. I would listen at
the door and wonder if we were all going
to live with Isabel, and if we would be
able to eat any more cake. When I saw
the redbrick building, I thought of Isabel.
I first saw it in the spring when my
daughter and I were driving to
Wilmington. I didn't mention it at first,
because it looked like a classic southern
building. But then it reappeared in the

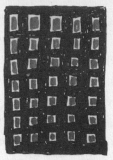

Zelda Grant's redbrick building.

next town, and the next day. I saw it all
along the highway. At first I was worried.
Not too worried, though, because I knew
it really wasn't there. I just wasn't sure
why I saw it so clearly. Then it began to
amuse me. I would look for it tucked
beyond a farm or a row of Main Street
shops. Honestly, it's very pretty, very
graceful architecturally. The landscape
would be much improved it they built a
few of them. I saw it for six or eight
months, but I haven't seen it in a while.

Rosa Garcia's Flowering Trees

They are beautiful, these flowers. Large
vibrant pink blooms, decorating trees
with no leaves, as if flowers always grew
in the wintertime. When I first saw
them, I loved them. *This isn't possible!* I

thought. It was autumn; there were leaves on the ground. We were on the train to Toronto. I watched these flowers for a while; then I turned to my friend Barbara and told her what I was seeing. I remember being quite enthusiastic, although I wasn't sure I should be saying so much. She just sort of stared at me. Then I made the mistake of telling her about the chain-link fences. I had been seeing chain-link fences everywhere. Well, many places they shouldn't be. They were okay. But the pink flowers were beautiful. Barbara just stared at me even harder. Then she asked a few questions about how long I had been seeing fences and flowers, and where

Rosa Garcia's flowering trees.

they appeared. She didn't seem any more comfortable with my answers. For some reason, though, I didn't really care. I just stopped telling people about them. You have to be careful what you say.

Buddy Burmester's Purple Flowers and Blackbirds

I see purple flowers in my bathroom sink, and sometimes on my pants, which is a little compromising. Since no one else sees them, though, I'm not so embarrassed. But can you imagine golf pants with purple flowers? I'd look like one of those hippies! I also see blackbirds. Powerful things, flying in sets of threes. My cousin

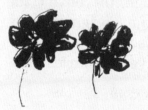

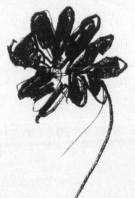

Buddy Burmester's purple flowers.

Harry has macular degeneration, too. He
sees frogs in his bathtub and a pretty
blond woman standing on his back porch,
which is very funny. Harry was never a
very successful ladies' man. My purple
flowers and blackbirds are not half as
interesting as frogs in the bathtub and a
woman on the back porch! I said to him,
"Harry, maybe she's a Radio City Music
Hall Rockette who made a detour
through New Jersey."

"Could be," he says. "She looks like a
Rockette is supposed to look. Too bad
she's not really there." You ought to talk
to Harry. He's not too unhappy about the
whole thing.

Mary Flannery and Dolly Kowalski both saw figures of people. Although they could not draw
these figures accurately enough to convey the
tangible reality with which they originally appeared, I've included their descriptions because
the figures are so representative of Charles Bonnet Syndrome.

Mary Flannery's Elizabethan Dinner Party

I was born in Belfast in 1928. My parents
died just before the war, so I went to live
in Boston with my Uncle Liam. My

mother, of course, never liked the British. But I always loved the theater and I loved Shakespeare. I used to dress up in my aunt's old dresses and pretend I was Juliet and Romeo was on his way over to the house. I don't think that has anything to do with my Elizabethan dinner party, though. That's what I call it. I see these very formal, earnest people sitting around my dining room table in full Elizabethan dress. Their outfits are made of bright, jeweled fabrics, with lots of lace, high collars, and pinched V-shaped waists. They look like they belong onstage or in the queen's court. They're not talkative, they don't seem hungry, and they don't seem upset. Actually, they appear to think it's perfectly natural to sit around my dining room table. They irritate me sometimes, but I think my mother would probably roll over in her grave.

Dolly Kowalski's Little Girls with Pink Bows

I see little girls with pink bows playing in my yard. At first, there was only one little girl. But after a while, she had several playmates. Now they come almost every evening for fifteen minutes or so and play with one another. They laugh and jump around. They are so delightful, so cheerful, so active. Their little white dresses and pink bows blow in the wind. I see them so incredibly clearly, much more clearly than I see anything else now. I enjoy seeing the details of their dresses and the expressions on their faces. I know that they aren't real, but you wouldn't believe how realistic they seem, how lively and pretty they are. I wish you could see them the way I do.

PART III:

Addressing AMD

CHAPTER 9

Why Visual Rehabilitation Is Right for You

You must do the thing you think you cannot do.
— **Eleanor Roosevelt**

When we begin to take our failures non-seriously, it means we are ceasing to be afraid of them. It is of immense importance to learn to laugh at ourselves.
— **Katherine Mansfield**

If you have any degree of vision loss or if you anticipate vision loss in the near future, visual rehabilitation is already right for you, because it empowers you with the skills and knowledge that will allow you to continue your life and make your own decisions about your future. However, Medicare will pay for services only when your vision is 20/70 or less, and many state and private agencies require vision of 20/200 or less. If you do not meet these minimums, you can still start your own visual rehabilitation by reading the chapters in this part of the book, learning their content, and adopting those elements you like. Early visual rehabilitation may have tremendous benefits, not the least of which is lowering your risk of depression with macular degeneration and ensuring a higher quality of life in the coming years.

What Does Visual Rehabilitation Include?

Visual rehabilitation is just like rehabilitation for any other kind of impairment. If you suffer a minor stroke that impairs the use of your right arm, you will receive occupational therapy. You'll be trained to do all the daily activities you need to do without relying heavily on that arm. Low vision affects at least as many daily activities as the loss of your right arm, so visual rehabilitation provides comparable training. Visual rehabilitation includes training in using your peripheral vision to read and training for daily activities. Visual rehabilitation also includes adapting your home with lighting, labels, and low-vision products. And it includes professional fitting for visual aids such as magnifiers and high-power lenses and training in their use. It may also include counseling and support groups. Since visual rehabilitation for adults is a relatively new field, programs vary in their scope and quality. Some places offer only visual aids; others offer more. That's why it's important to locate all of the services for which you are eligible so that you have the best experience.

Visual Rehabilitation Is Not Resignation

Sometimes people fear that if they pursue visual rehabilitation, they're resigning themselves to low vision, giving up on a possible cure, and giving up on their future. But visual rehabilitation is not about resignation. It's about figuring out what you would enjoy doing, pursuing it with whatever means are available, learning new skills, and letting self-judgment go. It's about having choices and influencing your life today. It's not about precluding choices that may be available tomorrow. Anyone pursuing visual rehabilitation can tell you that it doesn't foster resignation—far from it. Visual rehabilitation at its best fosters courage—the courage to try new things and keep your sense of humor. It fosters commitment—the willingness to stick with it and do the most you can. And visual rehabilitation fosters confidence—the belief that you can do more than you think you can. Right here, right now. And you can!

Finding a Visual Rehabilitation Program in Your Area

If there is a rehabilitation program in your area, be sure to go. They will provide invaluable hands-on training and additional resources or advice. To find a program in your area, follow the steps outlined in appendix A. If there is no program in your area, the Rehabilitation Workshop in this book is designed to be your personal home version of our program here in Michigan. You can also use this book as a supplement to another program or to appointments with a low-vision optometrist who can fit you with optical aids.

YOUR HOME VISUAL REHABILITATION PROGRAM

Your home rehabilitation program includes five chapters, each covering a different topic: lighting; reading with low vision; magnifiers, telescopes, and computers; driving, transportation alternatives, and traveling; and adapting your home and interacting with the community. Although each chapter can be understood independently, the chapters were written to build upon one another. As a result, each chapter assumes that you know the information covered in the previous one. For example, chapter 14, which talks about adaptations you can make to your home, assumes that you already know about the lighting information covered in chapter 10 and the magnifier information covered in chapter 12. For this reason, it's best to proceed through each chapter in the order in which they are presented. This is particularly true for chapter 11, "Your Reading Workshop," which must be followed exactly as presented. You may also want to order the free low-vision product catalogs listed in appendix C and browse through them as you work through the program.

Working with a Family Member or Friend

Most of this rehabilitation program doesn't directly call for assistance from friends or family. However, many suggestions do assume that you have someone who can lend a helping hand, especially with things like rearranging furniture, buying and installing new lighting fixtures, and learning the bus system. The Reading Workshop in chapter 11 also requires a partner. You may want to skim through the whole program first with a friend or family member to determine which parts you already know, which you may be able to do on your own or with minimal assistance, and which parts will take more time. You may already have one family member or friend who can serve as a partner for the whole program. If not, consider asking several different people to each help with a small portion. To accommodate everyone's schedules, consider setting up dates in advance for reading chapters or working on different tasks or tips. This approach may be particularly helpful for the Reading Workshop, which requires mastering several different separate lessons. Working

with friends or family members on visual rehabilitation can also make the program more enjoyable. And they'll learn a lot, too. In fact, there
are several tips for friends and family along
the way.

SUPPLIES FOR CHAPTER 11: "YOUR READING WORKSHOP"

- 1 thick black felt-tip pen

- 1 package of at least sixty plain white
  three-by-five index cards

- 1 package of ready-made stick-on
  (sticky) black letters 1–1½ inches
  high. Sticky letters are available at
  most office supply shops. If you cannot
  find them, you can use your black felt-
  tip marking pens to print individual
  letters.

- 5–10 pages of an article from your
  favorite magazine or a book chapter
  enlarged on a quality copier with
  sharp black ink on white paper just
  large enough so that you can read the
  words.

SUPPLIES FOR CHAPTER 14: "SAVING SIGHT AT HOME AND IN YOUR COMMUNITY"

- 1 medium-width black permanent marker

- 1 package of large rubber bands

- 1 small package of safety pins

- Large black, white, and bright neon orange stickers

- Ready-made stick-on (sticky) black letters 1–2 inches high, or higher if they are more easily readable

- 1 tube each of black, white, and orange puff paint. Puff paint is available at many fabric stores and is sometimes marketed as fabric or T-shirt paint. You can squeeze it onto fabric, metal, or other surfaces for labeling. Since it dries slightly puffy, you can also feel it.

Supplies to Purchase and Have Handy

Chapter 11, "Your Reading Workshop," and chapter 14, "Saving Sight at Home and in Your

Community," both call for a small collection of inexpensive supplies. You can find almost everything on both of these lists at a local office supply store. You may want to collect them before you begin your rehabilitation program.

Supplies to Gather for Yourself

Now that you are starting your visual rehabilitation program and purchasing the supplies you need for various chapters, don't forget the most important supplies of all: the ones you need for you. Visual rehabilitation can make living easier, but it does take some determination and courage. And like all things worth having in life, it takes some work and some humor, too. You've got all the skills and qualities you'll need—but gathering them together as you start your program and keeping them at your fingertips will help you have a positive, empowering experience. Remember, you do have choices. You can influence the quality of your life. Beginning a visual rehabilitation program and committing to living fully in the world in whatever way is best for you are choices to positively influence the quality of your life. You can do it. I know you can.

SUPPLIES FOR YOU:
THE THREE C'S

- **Courage:** trying new things and keeping your sense of humor

- **Commitment:** sticking with it and doing the most you can

- **Confidence:** believing you can do more than you think you can

CHAPTER 10

Making Things Brighter: Lighting

I never knew a lightbulb could make such a difference.
—Edina Williams

Lighting goes with *everything*. Doing something? You need good light. That's the bottom line. But it's surprising how little we actually think about light or realize that we can dramatically change the lighting in our own home. Every week occupational therapist Annie Riddering and I meet people who don't realize that they need more light now than they used to. "One new patient sent me back to the office when I arrived at her house for a rehabilitation appointment," Annie told me recently. "We had talked the week before over the phone, and she listened to everything I said about light. When I arrived for our appointment, she greeted me with a big smile and said, 'Annie! You're not going to believe this, but I changed every lightbulb in my house and now I'm seeing things I haven't seen in a year.'" Another patient, to her amazement, found herself able to read print twice as small as she usually could by using the directed light of a gooseneck desk lamp. Not all problems can be solved so easily, but increasing lighting and reducing glare will help tremendously.

Reducing Glare

If you have macular degeneration, you may be sensitive to glare, especially from fluorescent lights or sunlight. This happens because macular degeneration may affect your eye's ability to modulate light. You can reduce glare by choosing softer light sources, like incandescent lights over fluorescent lights, or by changing your position in relationship to the light source. For example, facing sunlight may be much less comfortable than facing away and allowing the sunlight to fall over your shoulder or come from the side if you are using a magnifier. Shiny book pages are often much more difficult to look at than matte finished pages. The same is true of highly polished furniture and floors; they can produce glare where carpeting, secured area rugs, and upholstered furniture would not. Reducing glare is an important component of good lighting in your home. If you are extremely glare-sensitive, you may choose to do some things, like dining at home or in restaurants, with less light than we recommend in this chapter. You may also choose to reduce the amount of sunlight in your home. As with every aspect of visual rehabilitation, the trick is to make the environment comfortable for you.

THE ONE-DAY OBSERVATION

You may already be aware of exactly when and where you need to add light or reduce glare in your home. But oftentimes we unconsciously adjust to low lighting without realizing that we are living with less light than we really need. Lighting conditions in our homes and our lighting needs also change depending upon the time of day and the type of activity we are pursuing. To help identify your home lighting conditions and lighting needs, take one day to observe lighting in your home by walking through it three times: once in the early morning, once in the afternoon, and once in the evening. If you live in an area with variable weather or seasons, you may want to observe your home more than once to see how changes in outdoor lighting affect your ability to see inside. Notice the following:

1. Which areas of your home have only medium or low lighting? Are your stairwells, porches, and closets adequately lit? Do you have bright, focused light in the areas where you do detailed work, like reading or cooking?

2. Which areas receive a great deal of sunlight and which do not? At which times of the day? How does your window dressing affect the amount of sunlight in your home?

3. Where does glare bother you? Is the glare from sunlight, light fixtures, or reflections?

4. During the same twelve-hour period, notice moments when you have trouble seeing. Ask yourself where you are sitting or standing when you find yourself frustrated. What are the lighting conditions?

Now that you have a more thorough understanding of the lighting conditions in your home and your particular lighting needs, you can use the information in the rest of this chapter to choose the changes that will be most effective for you.

IMPROVING LIGHTING IN YOUR HOME

Lighting is very personal. What works for one person may not work for another, so you may have to experiment a bit with furniture arrangements, window dressings, fixtures, and lightbulbs to find the combination that works best for you. The next few sections outline lighting options. A list of the most popular suggestions for people with macular degeneration follows.

Using Sunlight in Your Home

While you are choosing new fixtures or bulbs or rearranging the lighting in your home, don't forget to use your free lighting—sunlight. Allow as much sunlight as you can into your home without tolerating too much glare. Sunlight is brighter and more powerful than artificial light. You can often see color contrasts or read better with sunlight than with lamps. If you do have bright afternoon light in your home, take your clothing choices for the following day to the sunniest room to make your selection, rather than choosing your clothing in the morning when your home is relatively dark. You may also want to rearrange your furniture or rooms to take advantage of the rhythms of sunlight. For example, if you like to drink coffee and do a crossword puzzle in the morning, you may be better off relaxing in a sunny bedroom than struggling to see in a sunless kitchen or living room. If you do sit in the sun, position your chair or couch with its back against the window so that the light falls on your page or coffee cup. You may also be better off replacing your heavy drapes with sheer curtains or blinds to allow as much sunlight as possible while reducing glare. Vertical blinds are an excellent option because then you can track the sun all day.

Light Fixture Options

There are essentially three categories of home light fixtures: fixed overhead lighting, inflexible floor or table lamps, and flexible desk lamps (gooseneck type or hinge type).

Overhead fixtures provide basic overall room light but are generally not adequate for detailed work. Inflexible floor or table lamps are also good for overall room light but do not always provide as much light as we assume they do. They tend to throw light toward the ceiling and the floor, providing only moderate to low light at eye level. Traditional shade lamps are the worst, since the shades mute most of the light and throw the rest all over the room. If your incandescent ceiling or floor fixtures aren't adequately lighting your rooms, try using at least 100-watt bulbs. For brighter light, you may consider a halogen pedestal lamp that sits on the floor (also called a torchère). Many people buy one for the room in which they spend the most time. Halogen lamps do have one serious drawback: they are very hot and can cause fires if they are knocked down on carpets or positioned too closely to drapes. For this reason, they are now sold with protective metal screens over the bulbs. Use them with caution.

For desk lamps, many people prefer halogen fixtures and bulbs because they are so bright. A 50-watt halogen reflector bulb gives light equivalent to a 150-watt incandescent bulb. However, some people find halogen desk lamps too hot. The most convenient fixture for detailed work is a gooseneck or hinge type adjustable table or floor lamp with an indoor floodlight bulb. They are particularly good if you are sensitive to glare, because you can position the light beam below the level of your eyes and still direct strong illumination onto a page or project. You can adjust the brightness of desk and floor lamps by moving them farther away, choosing fixtures with dimmers, or changing lightbulbs.

Lightbulb Options

There are four different types of lightbulbs available at hardware stores and superstores and through low-vision catalogs: fluorescent, halogen, chromalux, and incandescent (incandescent bulbs come in two models: regular or floodlight). Each type has advantages and disadvantages.

Fluorescent and halogen bulbs provide the brightest light, which many people appreciate, but they do have some drawbacks. Fluorescent bulbs can only be used in fixtures designed for them; they also tend to cause glare, which can be extremely irritating. Halogen bulbs cause less glare but tend to be more expensive, and they are sometimes too bright, too hot, or too heavy for desk lamps. For these reasons, halogen bulbs are best used in pedestal floor lamps. Traditional halogen bulbs fit only in halogen lamps, but halogen reflector bulbs do have standard bases that can fit any lamp.

Chromalux and incandescent bulbs are somewhat similar. Chromalux bulbs are available in 60- and 100-watt frosted glass; they are designed to imitate natural light and are cooler than ordinary incandescent bulbs. Incandescent bulbs, which are the familiar regular lightbulbs, are cheaper and more widely available. In higher wattages, however, they tend to be hot and are not quite as bright as fluorescent or halogen. For this reason, incandescent indoor floodlight bulbs are very popular with people who have macular degeneration because they provide brighter, more focused light without adding more wattage or heat. We often find that they are the best bulbs of all.

CAUTION

When you purchase new fixtures, make sure that your electrical system can handle any extra wattage. When you use stronger bulbs in new or existing fixtures, make sure you follow the manufacturer's instructions. Using the wrong lightbulb in a fixture can ruin your fixture and short your entire electrical system.

Popular Suggestions for Increasing Light

- Replace your incandescent lightbulbs that are less than 75 to 100 watts with 75- to 100-watt bulbs. For detailed work, use a 45- or 65-watt incandescent indoor floodlight or a halogen reflector bulb.

- Buy a small, inexpensive gooseneck or hinge type lamp with an indoor floodlight bulb. Make sure it is easy to carry and adjust. Take this lamp with you around the house to places where you most frequently need light for detailed work, such as reading or setting laundry dials. Perch it on tabletops, sinks, counters, appliances, or desks. In the areas where you use it most frequently, consider purchasing one to place there permanently. You can find models for ten to twenty-five dollars at local hardware stores or superstores that sit on any surface, screw into walls, or clip onto desktops or bed frames.

- Buy a bright lightweight flashlight or penlight. Make sure it is not too heavy. Carry it in your pocket or purse. Use it to read labels in the grocery store and menus in restaurants, and to see things around your house, such as clothes in the closet, stove dials, alarm systems, thermostats, and cleaning fluid bottles in the garage. Camping stores are often the best sources for strong lightweight flashlights.

Popular Suggestions for Reducing Glare

- Replace irritating fluorescent lights with incandescent light fixtures. Use at least 75- to 100-watt incandescent bulbs, indoor floodlight bulbs, or chromalux bulbs.

- Cover Formica countertops, glass tables, or shiny polished wood tables with tablecloths or towels. Cover polished hardwood floors or tile floors that reflect glare with heavy area rugs. Make sure you secure all rugs so they do not slide and you do not trip on their edges. Move mirrors that reflect glare.

- Use venetian blinds or, better yet, sheer curtains to reduce sun glare while allowing as much sunlight as possible into your home.

- To reduce unavoidable glare in your home, grocery stores, and restaurants, wear a pair of light yellow or plum NOIR (wraparound) glasses. These glasses can be worn alone or over your prescription glasses. They are available through the low-vision catalogs listed in appendix C for fifteen to twenty dollars.

- To reduce glare outside, wear a pair of blue-blocker sunglasses or add blue blockers to your existing sunglasses or regular glasses or wear a pair of dark yellow NOIR glasses either by themselves or over your regular glasses. Blue blockers will increase the tint of your lenses and cut glare, but they will not decrease the overall amount of light you perceive. In other words, unlike regular sunglasses, they will not make the world look darker. Talk to your optician about these options, and see chapter 3 for more information on blue blockers.

LIGHTING IN PUBLIC PLACES

Unfortunately, we often get too much sunlight outside and too little inside. Many restaurants keep their lighting low to create ambience, while grocery stores blast fluorescent lights to highlight their products. So what can you do? Keep a pair of lightly tinted wraparound glasses with you to reduce indoor glare (see Popular Suggestions for Reducing Glare) and carry a small flashlight or penlight for reading print or identifying objects in poorly lit stores and restaurants. When you dine out, request a table with good lighting or one near a sunny window. Sit with your back to the window so that the sunlight falls on the menu and on your plate. If you find a restaurant with particularly good lighting and a friendly staff, compliment them and give them your business. Restaurants need to know that low lighting and fluorescent lighting can be extremely inconvenient for their customers and can discourage seniors from returning. Remember, you aren't alone. There are more than 1.5 million Americans with advanced macular degeneration who need more light to see. They like to dine out, too.

CHAPTER 11

Your Reading Workshop

That which we persist in doing becomes easier to do, not that the nature of the task has changed, but our ability to do it has increased.
—Ralph Waldo Emerson

We often think of reading as a skill that we learned years ago in grade school. Now we simply know how to read. But reading is actually more like playing tennis: It's very practice-sensitive. Just as your tennis game improves with practice, so your reading ability improves with practice, too. As a rule, the more we read, the more efficiently we can read. This is true of everyone, especially everyone with low vision. And it's true of all kinds of reading, not just reading novels or articles but reading signs and labels, too. If you haven't been reading for a while because of low vision, you may not be able to read as much as you actually could with training and practice. The Reading Workshop will teach you new techniques for reading with low vision and help you practice them. Even if you aren't interested in reading, reading practice will make it easier to identify packages in the grocery store, see food at the table, crochet, or walk down the sidewalk, because reading practice trains you to use the clearest areas of your remaining vision most effectively.

Magnifiers and the Reading Workshop

There is another great reason to complete the Reading Workshop: many people find that it enables them to use weaker magnifiers, sometimes magnifiers as much as two or three times (X powers) weaker. This is good because weaker magnifiers are usually easier to use than stronger ones. They cover a wider area of print, and you can hold them farther from your eyes, so they give you a more comfortable reading distance.

Lighting and the Reading Workshop

Really good lighting is absolutely necessary for the Reading Workshop. In fact, good lighting is necessary whenever you read. You will not be able to do the exercises in this chapter without good lighting. I recommend a gooseneck or adjustable table or floor lamp with an indoor floodlight bulb. Adjust the lamp so it shines directly on the exercise or reading material. Do not use a regular incandescent lightbulb that is less than 100 watts or lamps with regular shades that do not shine light directly on the material. Overhead lighting, no matter how bright, may not be sufficient, especially if you lean over while you read, casting shadows on the material.

Inside Your Reading Workshop

Anne T. Riddering, M.S., O.T.R., the director of occupational therapy at our visual rehabilitation program in Michigan, designed this Reading Workshop especially for you to use at home. It's almost the same one she uses here with our patients. The workshop has three exercises. You must complete all three exercises in the order in which they appear.

The first exercise, "Finding Your Scotoma," takes about an hour. Annie usually does this exercise with our patients in their homes. You will need an "Annie," too: a friend or family member who can work with you. In this exercise you will find the weakest area of your central vision and practice moving it out of the way in order to see clearly.

The second exercise, "Relearning to Read," may take anywhere from a few hours to several days. In this exercise you will relearn which letters of the alphabet look alike, making it easier for you to quickly identify a misleading letter when you encounter it. Annie spends time with our patients on this one, too—so you may want your friend or family member to help.

The third exercise, "Reading Practice," is an extended reading practice program you can do on

your own that will take one hour a day for two to
four weeks.

Confidence, Commitment, and Courage

Ah! you may be thinking. *This is going to take
some effort.* And you're right. It will. But it'll be
worth the effort. You may find the workshop enjoyable and fairly easy. Or you may find it challenging. But you can do it, and it will help you to
read print and to see just about anything else
more effectively. Gather your confidence, commitment, and courage, and set them next to you. Be
determined, but be kind to yourself, too. Stick
with the exercises. Take breaks when you're tired
or frustrated. Be sure to give yourself rewards for

DO NOT USE MAGNIFIERS FOR THE READING WORKSHOP

Do not use your magnifiers for any
part of the Reading Workshop,
including Reading Practice. Wear your
regular reading glasses or no glasses
at all if you read better without them.
Magnifiers come later, in chapter 12.

---

trying. If you have a hard time working alone, ask someone to do the workshop with you. And don't worry about your pace. Remember, it was the tortoise who won the race in Aesop's fable, not the hare. You can do it. Go for it!

GETTING STARTED: WORKSHOP MATERIALS

Collect the Following Materials:

- 1 "Annie" (family member or friend who can be your partner for the first exercise and perhaps the second, too). Read through this chapter with your partner to get a sense of how much time you may need together.

- 1 package of fifty-two plain, unlined white three-by-five-inch index cards.

- 1 package of ready-made stick-on black letters 1–1½ inches high.

Make sure you have the entire alphabet in both capital and lowercase letters. You can find stick-on letters at many office supply stores, drugstores, and superstores and in low-vision catalogs. If these letters are not available, you can use a thick black felt-tip marker to print your own.

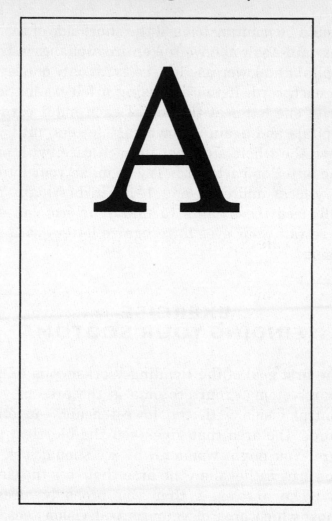

Preparing the Materials

Place one ready-made stick-on letter lengthwise at the top of each index card—the top of the letter should be pointing toward the short side of the index card—so you have the entire alphabet in both capital and lowercase letters, with only one letter on each card. If you are using a felt-tip marker, write one letter at the top of each index card in capitals and again in lowercase letters until you have the whole alphabet in each case, with only one letter on each card. Try to make your letters very clear and even and 1–1½ inches high. You will need these cards to find your scotoma and to retrain your eyes to recognize letters with low vision.

EXERCISE I:
FINDING YOUR SCOTOMA

The first goal of the Reading Workshop is to find your scotoma. Your scotoma is the area of your central vision with the lowest acuity—in other words, the area that gives you the blurriest picture. You might wonder why we should look for this area rather than the area that sees the clearest. The answer is that you probably already know which area of your central vision sees the clearest, even if you aren't aware that you know. Most people automatically adjust to low vision by moving their eyes when they look at an object so they can see it with the area of their central vision that provides the clearest view. However, most people are not aware of which area or areas provide the blurriest view. If you know which area provides the blurriest view and you learn to move it out of the way, you will have covered both of your bases. You'll naturally look at things with the best area of your vision. And if that doesn't automatically work, you'll also know how to move the worst part of your vision out of the way in order to produce the clearest view.

Ring Scotomas and Multiple Scotomas

Most people's scotoma is close to the center of their vision, so that the clearest areas of their vision will be farther out around the edges. You may have only one scotoma, especially if you have relatively good vision, although some people have more than one. If you have multiple scotomas, focus on finding the blurriest one. About 20 percent of people with macular degeneration have a ring scotoma, which is a scotoma that forms a ring around your central vision, leaving a small, clearer area in the middle. This means that you may see things fairly clearly, but you also may lose the image quickly if you move your eye slightly. If you have a ring scotoma, practicing keeping your eye directly on whatever you wish to see and moving your scotoma out of the way when necessary will be very helpful.

Finding Your Scotoma

Our natural instinct is to move our eyes toward any object we want to see. To find your scotoma, however, you must keep your eyes on your partner's nose throughout the exercise. Read all seven steps first so you understand the whole exercise, and then begin with the first.

Step 1

Position two chairs facing each other so that their seats are a foot or so apart. Hardback or kitchen chairs may be easiest to maneuver. Sit facing your partner so your knees are nearly touching. Don't wear your glasses, unless you absolutely cannot do the exercise without them. Do not use any magnifiers.

Step 2

Look at your partner's nose. If you cannot see his or her nose, look directly at the spot where you know the nose should be. Do not move your eyes during the exercise. Your partner should watch your eyes to make sure you are always looking at his or her nose.

Step 3

Your partner selects a card with a capital letter and holds the card up facing you, so that it is halfway between the two of you, at the same height as the top of your forehead. If your face were a clock, your partner would be holding the card at twelve o'clock.

Step 4

Try to identify the letter.

Step 5

Your partner selects another card and holds it in the one o'clock position. Try to identify this new letter. Continue around all twelve points of the clock, with a new letter for each point. Finally, your partner selects yet another letter and places it in the center of the clock, moving it a few inches up, down, to the right, and to the left. Identify the letter.

Step 6

As you go around the clock, you and your partner should notice the position in which the letter is hardest to identify or disappears altogether. This is where your scotoma is.

Step 7

Confirm and remember the location of your scotoma by double-checking it. Your partner selects another letter and holds it where you can see it, then moves it into your scotoma so that it disappears or becomes blurry. Repeat this until you are sure you know where your scotoma is.

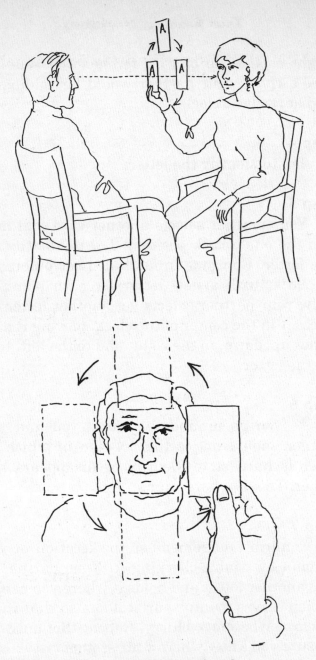

Illustrations of reading exercise I.

What If I Don't Find My Scotoma?

If you don't find your scotoma, don't worry, especially if you know you have pretty good vision. Your scotoma is probably very small. However, you may want to double-check the following possibilities and try the exercise again:

- Make sure you are looking at your partner's nose at all times. You may be moving your eyes to avoid your scotoma when you look at the letter.

- Make sure you aren't reading the letter before your partner puts it in a test position. Sometimes if you already know what the letter is, your brain will automatically fill in the image, making it look clearer than it is.

- Use lowercase letters or smaller sticky letters or print smaller letters on additional index cards and use them instead. Capital letters may be too large to catch your scotoma.

What If My Scotoma Seems to Be Everywhere?

If your scotoma seems to be everywhere, double-check the following possibilities and try the exercise again:

- You may not have enough well-directed light in the room. Add lighting or move to a brighter area.

- Your partner may be holding the card too far out to the side or too close to his or her own nose. Have your partner adjust his or her placement of the card.

- The letters on the card may be too small for you to read. Print a larger letter on a card with a thick black marker. Repeat the exercise using the larger letter.

If your scotoma still seems to be everywhere and you have moderate to very low vision (20/150 or higher), you may have a complicated scotoma pattern. Ideally, you should go to a low-vision rehabilitation program that has a scanning laser ophthalmoscope (SLO). The SLO can photograph your scotoma pattern so your doctor knows exactly where your best areas of vision are. You can call the national organizations listed in the back of the book for references or ask your doctor for a referral. If the program you find does not have an SLO, go anyway. They will be able to help you find your scotoma and fit you correctly with magnifiers, as well as provide training in their use. If you can't find a program, don't worry. You can still benefit from the rest of the Reading Workshop.

Practice Moving Your Scotoma

You can move your scotoma out of the way by moving your eye toward it. This may seem counterintuitive at first, but try it until you're comfortable. Whenever you are reading and you have particular trouble, try moving your scotoma out of the way by moving your eye toward it. This may take some practice, which you can do along with exercises 2 and 3, but once you can do so easily, it will help your reading a great deal.

EXERCISE 2:
RELEARNING TO READ

When we learned to read in grade school we had to memorize each letter of the alphabet. It was a challenging task at the time because the letters look a lot alike. By now, though, we're so used to them that we don't realize how confusing they can be. More important, we don't realize that they are confusing in a predictable way. Since certain letters look alike, we will almost always confuse them with each other, rather than with letters that look significantly different. In order to read efficiently with low vision, you need to relearn what you first learned in grade school: which letters you are likely to confuse. When you have this information at your fingertips, you can quickly double-check a letter by considering the logical alternatives.

Don't be discouraged by the number of letters involved in this exercise. Make a game of it; take them one group at a time. Everyone has difficulties remembering them at first, but you can do it! It just takes patience and practice.

Relearning Capital Letters

Begin with capital letters and do not continue to the lowercase letters until you feel confident that you have memorized the capitals. Trying to do too many letters at once can be overwhelming. Go through all five steps without worrying about remembering every letter the first time around. This will give you an understanding of the whole exercise. Once you have gone through all five steps, try to memorize the letter groups. Test yourself with your index cards once a day until you know the letter groups by heart. Notice which letters are most confusing to you and pay special attention to them.

Step 1: The Two X's

Take out your **X** and **K** and put them on the table next to each other. Now cover the left side of each letter and you will see that the right sides are almost identical. So, when you see what you think is either an **X** or a **K**, be sure to double-check the left side of the letter to tell the difference.

Step 2: The Four Straight Arrows

Take out **I**, **T**, **J**, and **L** and put them on the table next to one another. Their straight lines make them look very similar, especially if the font in which they are printed doesn't exaggerate their differences.

Step 3: The Four Round Ones

Take out your **C**, **G**, **O**, and **Q** and put them on the table next to one another. Notice that they all share identical left sides. If you cover the right side of each letter, they look the same. So when you see one of these four letters, remember to double-check the right side of the letter to tell the differences.

And Their Flat-Sided Cousins

Leave the **O** on the table and put **D** and **U** next to it. Notice that if the tops were gone, they would look almost like triplets. If you think you see one of these three letters, double-check the top of the letter to tell the difference.

Step 4: The Five Straight-Round Combos

Take out **E** and **F** and put them next to each other. Then take out **B**, **P**, and **R** and put them next to one another. Cover the bottom right corners of **E** and **F** and you'll see that they look alike. Then cover the bottom right corners of **B**, **P**, and **R**, and they'll look the same, too. **B** can also sometimes look like **S**. Now cover the right sides of **F**, **P**, and **R** and they'll look alike.

Step 5: The Five Diagonal Devils

These letters are the toughest of all. Take out the **N**, **M**, **W**, **V**, and **Y** and put them next to one another. You will see that they are all combinations of straight and diagonal lines, which can be very confusing. To tell them apart, look carefully at the bottoms of the letters.

Congratulations!
You're halfway there.
Don't give up!

REVIEWING AND REMEMBERING CAPITAL LETTERS

The Two X's:	X, K
The Four Straight Arrows:	I, T, J, L
The Four Round Ones:	C, G, O, Q
Their Flat-Sided Cousins:	D, U
The Five Straight-Round Combos:	E, F, B, P, R
The Five Diagonal Devils:	N, M, W, V, Y

Relearning Lowercase Letters

Step 1: The Two Dots and Two Crosses and the L

Take out the **i**, **j**, and **l**. To tell them apart, you need to look at the top of the letter to see if there is a dot and the bottom to see whether or not the letter is an **i** or a **j**. Now leave the **l** on the table and place it next to the **f** and **t**. As with the dots, you need to look at the top of the letter to double-check the cross and then see if there is a curl indicating an **f**. Of course, if there is no dot and no cross, you always have an **l**.

Step 2: The Little Round Vowels

Take out the **c**, **e**, **o**, and **a** (some forms of **a** are entirely round, resembling an **o**). To tell these letters apart, you need to look at their right sides.

Step 3: One Hump or Two, or Is It a U?

Take out **m**, **n**, and **u**. These three are nearly identical triplets when they're buried in the middle of a word. You can tell them apart if you make a point of looking at the top of the letter where you can see if it's open or closed and how many humps it has.

Step 4: The Pot Bellies and Straight Backs

Take out the **b**, **d**, **h**, and **p** and set them next to one another. These are the pot bellies and straight backs. They can be confusing because they all have a stem and some form of roundness that may be open or closed at the bottom. When you come across any of these letters, be sure to look first at the top and then at the bottom to double-check the stems and openings of the letters. This strategy of double-checking stems and openings will also help you with **h**, **n**, and **r**. In some fonts **g**, **p**, and **q** also look similar.

Step 5: Diagonal Devils Revisited

Take out **v**, **w**, and **y**. These three letters are just as likely to be confused in lowercase as they are in their uppercase forms. To tell the difference, look at the bottom to check for the stem of the **y** and then look at the top to check the number of points to tell if it's either a **v** or a **w**.

REVIEWING AND REMEMBERING THE LOWERCASE LETTERS

The Two Dots and	i, j, l and
Two Crosses and the **L**:	f, t, l
The Little Round Vowels:	c, e, o, a
One Hump or Two, or Is It a **U**?:	m, n, u
The Pot Bellies and	b, d, h, p,
Straight Backs:	h, n, r
	and g, p, q
The Diagonal Devils Revisited:	v, w, y

Congratulations!
You've done it!
Great job!

EXERCISE 3: READING PRACTICE

Now you can apply the skills you've learned from exercises 1 and 2 to reading. Take out your five to ten enlarged photocopied pages (see "Supplies for Chapter 11: 'Your Reading Workshop' " in chapter 9). Begin practicing with these pages. Read them continually for at least fifteen minutes at a time, three times a day, for a week. When this becomes easy, copy another set of the pages from the book in the smallest print size you can read without straining and without using glasses or magnifiers. If you use print that is too large, you won't be challenged to use your new reading skills. If you use print that is too small, you will tire and become too frustrated to really use your new reading skills. Continue reading three times a day for one week and moving down to the next smaller print size if the reading becomes too easy. When you have reached the smallest print size that you can read, practice with that size for one more week. Remember to have good lighting for reading of any kind, including practices (see chapter 10 for lighting advice).

ADDITIONAL SKILLS: AUDIO READING AND BRAILLE READING

I call listening to magazines or books on tape audio reading because it is another form of reading, alongside standard and large-print reading and Braille reading. To have the widest access to entertainment and information and the most flexible skill set to do whatever you'd like to do, learn as many ways of reading as you can.

Audio Reading

At first glance, audio reading doesn't look like a new skill. Of course we already know how to listen to a tape-recorded book or magazine. You just pop the tape into the machine, right? Not exactly. Audio reading is a skill, too. It takes learning to operate the player easily and adjust the volume and pace, and it takes learning to visualize. We are often so reliant on seeing words to trigger our imaginations or remember information that we haven't exercised our powers of listening. Often it takes some adjustment and practice to fully enjoy the pleasure of listening to recordings—but if we take the time, they open up worlds to us. Be sure to enroll in the NLS (for Americans) or CNIB (for Canadians) national library programs (see appendixes B and F, respectively) and subscribe to the many other programs that provide free magazines, newspaper articles, and books on tape. Listening is reading—and it's a skill, too.

Braille Reading

Braille has gotten a bad rap among those of us who didn't grow up reading it. While learning Braille requires patience, memorization, and some tactile sensitivity in your fingertips, it's not as hard as people say, and it can be both useful and freeing (just think: no worries about lighting or magnification). You can use Braille not only to read poetry or books but also to label items in your home. The Hadley School for the Blind offers free correspondence courses for people with vision loss and their family members and friends. The school was founded by Dr. William Hadley in 1920 after he lost his sight at age fifty-five and discovered that there were very few Braille classes for adults. To find out about the Hadley School programs, see their listing in appendix B.

CHAPTER 12

Making Things Bigger: Magnifiers, Telescopes, and Computers

As we go about our daily activities, let us maintain a positive attitude, knowing full well that there are more sophisticated devices constantly being made available to us to help in daily living.

—Bert Silverman
AMD patient
and author of *Bert's Eye View:*
Coping with Macular Degeneration

Magnifiers are fantastic tools. You can do all kinds of things with magnifiers that aren't possible without them. But magnifiers are also tricky. My patients often tell me that their thoughtful son or daughter gave them a perfectly good magnifier for their birthday and it doesn't work at all. Technically, magnifiers always work. Their job is to magnify and they always do. But magnifiers are made in different powers and styles, and they magnify clearly only when they are held at the correct distance from an object. You have to choose magnifiers with the right power for your visual acuity, you have to choose the right styles for your needs, you have to use your magnifier correctly, and you have to have adequate lighting. Since magnifiers are rarely sold with purchasing instructions or users' manuals, it's very easy to get the wrong one if you're choosing your own. And it's true that the wrong magnifier will not work for you.

MAGNIFIERS

More Expensive Is Not Always Better

Magnifiers vary tremendously not only in power but also in style and price. There are different kinds of magnifiers for reading, for doing detailed work with both hands, for distance viewing, and for walking around. Magnifiers come in many sizes, shapes, and weights. They come attached to various handles, stands, headbands, neck cords, and jewelry chains. Some require you to hold them steady; others don't. They cost anywhere from $10 to $2,000 or more, especially if you consider lamp magnifiers, electronic magnifiers, or computer magnifying systems. More expensive, however, does not always mean better. On the one hand, if you have pretty good vision and you want to read the newspaper, a $350 high-tech lamp may be less useful to you than a $10 goose-neck desk lamp with an indoor floodlight bulb and a $35 paperweight magnifier. On the other hand, if you have less than 20/400 vision, the absolute best magnifier for reading anything will be a video magnifier, also called a closed-circuit television (CCTV). The bottom line is that the right magnifier for you is the one that enables you to do exactly what you want with the greatest ease.

How Much Money Can You Expect to Spend?

You probably need at least three or four magnifiers: a portable hand magnifier for spot reading, a stand magnifier for continuous reading, a head-mounted magnifier for doing a task with both hands, and possibly a distance magnifier. These basic magnifiers cost between $10 and $120, so you can purchase four magnifiers for the price of one high-quality pair of bifocals. You may choose to buy more expensive models or buy more than four, but you can have at least a basic set for about $200 to $300. The exception to this is the video magnifier (CCTV), which is an excellent tool for anyone with less than 20/70 vision. If you have less than 20/400 vision you should definitely consider purchasing one. CCTVs use a small video camera that magnifies any type of print, picture, or small object onto a television screen. They range in price from about $250 to

$2,500 depending on the type of model and its features. Check with your low-vision program or local retailer of low-vision supplies or the catalogs of the companies listed in appendix C for the latest information on CCTVs.

Testing and Returning Magnifiers

Do not buy a magnifier without a return guarantee. You don't want to be stuck with one that doesn't work for you. Reputable catalogs, programs, and dealers will offer you a wide choice

---

GOOD ADVICE

Talk to your doctor before you purchase any optical aid that costs more than $500, unless you are purchasing a CCTV. Magnifiers, high-power lenses, special glasses, and standard telescopes should not be more expensive than a designer pair of glasses. They are often less. Call a low-vision program in your area for help with these choices. Call the organizations listed in appendix A for help with finding a program.

---

and a free trial period or a full refund within thirty days (except for computer software, which is usually not returnable because it is so easily copied). At Low Vision Living, we loan magnifiers we feel are right for testing at home, often providing several models so that people can compare and choose the particular style that works best for them. Many sales representatives for CCTVs will deliver the equipment to you for testing at no cost, and some offer a one-month rental, the fee for which can be applied to the purchase price. Remember to test your magnifiers as soon as you receive them. Return unwanted ones in their original packaging so they can be resold.

Choosing the Right Strength

DIOPTERS AND X POWERS

The first thing to know about buying magnifiers, especially those for seeing up close, is that you shouldn't buy one without knowing what power you need. The power of a magnifier indicates the strength of its lens. It is like a prescription in regular eyeglasses, although prescriptions are much more specific. Nevertheless, just as you need to get glasses with the right prescription, you need to get magnifiers in the right power for them to be useful.

The strength of magnifying lenses is measured in both diopter powers and X powers; some products use diopter powers and others use

X powers. For example, most reading glasses are advertised in diopter powers. Diopter powers are written as "+ some number." You may see reading glasses in drugstores and catalogs labeled +1 or +2, meaning that they are 1 or 2 diopters in strength. Most magnifiers are advertised in X powers, which are written as "some number X." You will see magnifiers labeled 3X, 4X, and so forth.

Diopter powers are the official scientific measurement of all lenses. In other words, all lenses have a certain diopter power. Diopter powers are therefore the most reliable and consistent measurement of strength across brands. So why do some brands use X powers instead? X powers became popular because they give us some practical information. X powers tell us roughly how many times larger a magnifier will make print or any object appear. So a 3X magnifier will magnify to three times the original size, if you hold the magnifier at the correct distance. X powers vary slightly across brands because they are calculated on either a U.S. or a European scale, depending on the manufacturer.

WHAT IS MY DIOPTER POWER OR X POWER?

If there is a rehabilitation program in your area, please go. They will help you select magnifiers and train you to use them. This is particularly critical for stronger magnifiers, since the higher the power, the trickier a magnifier is to use. If there is no program in your area, *Macular Degeneration's* Magnifier Selection Chart is designed for you. You can use it to determine your power by the print size you can read. Turn to the chart and follow these four steps:

1. Wear your usual reading glasses and sit in a well-lit area.

2. Hold the Selection Chart 16 inches (40 cm) away.

3. Choose the smallest line you can read comfortably, without straining.

4. Follow the print line across the page to the four columns on the right.

The first two columns tell you what power magnifier you will probably need, measured in both U.S. and European X powers. The third column tells you what power reading glasses you will need, measured in diopters. The fourth column gives the visual acuity that usually matches these particular powers. The last column is only there to provide out-of-town family and friends with a ballpark guesstimate of the magnifier strength you need. For example, if they know that your vision is 20/80, they can order a magnifier for you in the corresponding X power.

WHEN POWERS VARY

Magnifier preferences vary among people. Two people who have exactly the same visual acuity measurements may prefer different-strength magnifiers. Why? Because the ease with which you read or do other tasks depends not only on your visual acuity but also on contrast sensitivity. If you have good contrast sensitivity (you can easily distinguish between objects of similar color or of similar lightness or darkness) you will not need as much magnification to read the same line of print as you would if you had less contrast sensitivity. In addition, practiced readers who have completed *Macular Degeneration*'s Reading Workshop or another visual rehabilitation reading program may not need quite as much magnification as those who do not read regularly and have no reading training.

Magnifier preferences may also vary for a single individual. For example, Dolores Lopez determined from *Macular Degeneration*'s Magnifier Selection Chart that 4X is her correct power. However, she bought a 4X lighted stand magnifier for reading at home and a 5X unlighted handheld model. Why? Without adequate light Dolores needs a more powerful magnifier. She carries the 5X unlighted model during the day to stores and restaurants that have variable lighting and finds that the 5X gives her enough additional magnification to compensate for less light.

Sample Print	Magnifier Powers		Diopters	Visual Acuity
	U.S.	European		
I can do this. It is very hard to do, but if I try my best I will succeed.			+2.5	20/30
I can do this. It is very hard to do, but I will try.	1.25X		+4–5	20/50
I can do this. It is very difficult.	1.75X	2.5X	+6–7	20/60
I can do this if I try.	2X	3X	+8	20/80
I can do this if I try.	3X	4X	+12	20/100

Sample Print	Magnifier Powers U.S.	European	Diopters	Visual Acuity
I can do this.	4X	5X	+16	20/125
I can do this.	5X	6X	+20	20/150
I can do this.	6X	7X	+24	20/200
I can do it.	7X	8X	+28	20/250

I can.   9X 10X   +36   20/300

I can.   12X 13X   +48   20/400

I will.   15X 16X   +60   20/500

Finally, magnifier powers vary slightly between catalogs because some catalogs list U.S. X powers and some list European X powers. Both are listed on the Magnifier Selection Chart. The chart serves as a guide for choosing the best-power magnifier for you, but you may find that you need a power higher or lower than you anticipated. Ordering magnifiers from a catalog is similar to ordering clothes from a catalog—it's not an exact science. If you have any questions, double-check your order with your ophthalmologist, optometrist, or catalog sales representative.

FINDING DIOPTERS AND POWERS FOR SOMEONE ELSE

If you are choosing a magnifier for a friend or family member who lives elsewhere or as a surprise gift, you will need to know the correct power or diopter magnifier to buy. If you don't have this information, you can use your friend or family member's 20/20-scale visual acuity measurement and the Magnifier Selection Chart to estimate the correct X power or diopter. If your friend or family member has been told by his or her eye doctor that his or her vision is "count fingers," this means it is less than 20/400. With 20/400 vision, you will need to buy at least a 12X or a +48 diopter magnifier or, better yet, contribute to the purchase of a CCTV. Always keep your receipt and the original packaging in case the magnifier needs to be returned or exchanged. If you have absolutely no information on your friend or family member's vision, buy another sort of product, such as a large-button high-contrast phone, talking calculator, or large-print address book. If your heart is set on a magnifier, try buying lightweight binoculars or opera glasses for distance viewing instead of a magnifier for close viewing.

Your Magnifier Toolbox

MAGNIFIERS AREN'T LIKE BIFOCALS

We're used to having just one pair of glasses to adjust our vision. Bifocals and trifocals, for example, are designed as all-in-one solutions. They're supposed to allow us to see anything at any distance. When you have low vision, though, you need much stronger magnification than a typical pair of bifocals will give you. Stronger lenses, though, do not come as all-in-one solutions. Magnifying lenses that enable you to see things up close, for example, are totally different from magnifying lenses that enable you to see things at a distance. It's the difference between microscopes and telescopes.

All magnifiers are tools, and the type of magnifier or tool you'll need depends on the type of task, how close you can hold the material, whether you need both your hands free, and how much contrast there is. Reading your mail requires a different tool from reading a sign across the street, since seeing the mail requires a lens that acts like a microscope and the sign requires a lens that acts like a telescope. There are lots of different magnifiers you can use to read print when you hold it quite close to your nose, but none of them will work for cooking meat in a pan (unless you plan to put your nose in with the meat, which we don't recommend!). There are also lots of different magnifiers you can hold to look at a price tag, but none of them will work for knitting or writing, because they don't allow you to use both your hands at the same time. Finally, the amount of magnification—and therefore the type of magnifier you can use—depends on the size of the object you want to see and whether it has low or high contrast. For example, knitting with a large pair of white needles and bright blue yarn requires less magnification than sewing the hem of navy blue pants with navy blue thread.

Tracy Williams, O.D., director of the nationally respected Deicke Center in Wheaton, Illinois, describes magnifiers as tools in a toolbox. Carpenters can't do their job with just a hammer. They also need a screwdriver, pliers, and probably a couple other tools, too. You may need a tool for reading your bills and letters at home, another for seeing price tags when you're out shopping, a third for knitting or writing, and a fourth— a telescope—for seeing your granddaughter in the school play or watching a football game. Which tools you choose depends on your eyesight, what you would like to do, and your personal preferences.

THREE TYPES OF MAGNIFIERS

Magnifiers are tools you use for seeing up close, something within arm's length of you, while telescopes are tools you use for seeing farther away, something across the room or across the street. There are essentially three types of magnifiers, each of which has its unique advantages and disadvantages:

1. Hands-free lenses that sit on your nose or your head

2. Handheld or hand-guided lenses

3. Video magnifiers or CCTVs

If you have fairly good vision, you will probably be able to use all three easily, which makes deciding between them a matter of personal preference. If you have lower vision, you may find that only certain models work well for you and you may vastly prefer the CCTV to any other magnification for reading bills, letters, other material.

I. Hands-Free Magnifiers

Hands-free magnifiers, as you might guess, leave your hands free to write or knit, for example, by sitting on your nose or head. They come as strong reading glasses, high-power clip-on lenses, and lenses mounted on headbands. The big disadvantage is that the stronger the lens, the closer you have to hold the material to the lens to see it. If the lens is on your nose, that means you have to hold whatever you want to see close to your nose.

For example, if you have normal vision and use bifocals, you can read a page fifteen to eighteen inches away. Doubling the power of your reading lens cuts this distance in half to seven or so inches, and tripling the power of the lens brings it to within a few inches of your nose. Some people prefer these strong lenses, but others find their close reading distance too uncomfortable. In this case, a CCTV is a better idea.

To gain a little distance between your eyes and the material, some companies have made lenses that clip onto your regular glasses and extend several inches out, like the Opticaid. Other models, such as the Opivisor and Magnifocuser, have lenses mounted on headbands. One of these, the Walters' Megaview, offers multiple interchangeable and combinable lenses for seeing at various close distances from a few inches to several feet away. The Beecher Mirage Telemicroscope and the Beecher KBK are more elaborate tools that focus at seventeen inches and can be used for computers and sheet music, for example.

High-power half-eye prism reading glasses are also available in low-vision catalogs and stores in powers up to +12 diopters. Prisms are built into the glasses so that you can hold material very, very close without looking cross-eyed. Full-size monocular reading glasses are also available in powers from +14 to +20 diopters. They are made with power in only one lens, for your best seeing eye, because they require you to hold material so close that you can't use both eyes even with prisms. These are very powerful lenses, so they're very tricky to fit and use correctly. When you're buying a magnifier this powerful, it's best to see a low-vision ophthalmologist or optometrist at your low-vision rehabilitation program so he or she can prescribe these lenses and help guide you in their use.

2. Handheld or Hand-Guided Magnifiers

These magnifiers are the familiar ones that we usually think of when we think of the word *magnifier*. You hold them with your hand above something you want to see, and if you have the right X power and hold them at the right distance—presto!—things look larger and clearer. There are actually three different types of hand-held magnifiers, which are useful for different tasks:

Hand Magnifiers for Spot Reading

Spot reading means reading something very briefly on the spot—like price tags or menus. These lenses come with handles or on pretty chains.

Many are lightweight and pocket-sized, and some come with built-in lights. There are lots of good models and brands available with different lens powers.

Stand Magnifiers for Continuous Reading

Stand magnifiers should actually be called sit magnifiers, since they literally sit on the page you are reading. Some look like Plexiglas paperweights or wedges, while others come with solid stands and built-in lights. Some models have interchangeable lenses of different powers. The paperweight type models work best for people who need little magnification (2X–3X). The lighted models work best for people who need anywhere from a little to a moderate amount of magnification (up to 5X–6X) and lots of light. If you need a great deal of magnification, a stand magnifier won't be strong enough and a CCTV is really your best bet for continuous reading. The advantage of a stand magnifier for reading is that you don't have to hold it and it automatically maintains a consistent distance from the page.

Hand and Stand Combo Magnifiers

If you need to use both your hands, you can get a combo magnifier that's mounted on a stationary arm. They work best for tasks like writing, knitting, and manicuring. They are less popular for continuous reading, since you have to move your page back and forth underneath the lens, which most people find annoyingly difficult. They may be mounted on gooseneck stands, with lamps attached, like the Big Eye, on immobile stands, or on a neck cord with a frame that rests on your chest. They're in the catalogs listed in appendix C, and lower-power models can sometimes be purchased in craft shops as well.

3. Video Magnifiers or CCTVs

CCTVs have revolutionized what people with visual impairments can do, and CCTV technology just keeps getting better and better. They're not supercheap, but they're amazingly useful for everyone and they can make a huge difference for anyone with moderate to severe vision loss. If you have less than 20/400 vision, a CCTV is the best option for reading anything at any time (except for computer software). CCTVs are also very popular with people who have better vision but prefer to have a large-screen view and a more comfortable reading distance than strong magnifiers allow.

CCTVs are electronic systems with a camera/projector and a screen. When you place a photograph, pill bottle, or printed page underneath the camera/projector, it beams the material onto a screen where it appears enlarged. CCTVs provide greater magnification and better contrast than any other type of magnification. They can show print and objects in both black-and-white and color, which is nice for viewing photos and magazine pictures and catalog shopping. There are two basic forms of CCTVs, and many models of each. See the low-vision catalogs in appendix C for the latest models and prices.

All-in-One Units

These models sit on your desk. They feature a monitor (like a TV or computer screen), below which there's a space to place whatever you'd like to view or use for writing or other activities, such as manicuring. All models have variable magnification and alternating black print on a white background or, for even higher contrast, white print on a black background. Color models are available as well. You control the degree of magnification and focus with levers, dials, or push buttons, depending on the model. The design may be important depending on your hand and wrist flexibility. They all have trays that lock in place for writing or are mobile for reading. My favorites are these: Telesensory's Aladdin and Aladdin Rainbow, Optolec's ClearView and Merlin, and MagniSight's Explorer.

Separate Camera Units

These units come without a screen and plug into your own TV, like a video game. The flick of a switch turns your TV into a reading machine and then back to a TV, as you wish. There is a wide variety of models in this category with many different features and prices from $300 to $3,000. The Max and Maxport by Enhanced Vision and the Magni-Cam and Primer by Innoventions are my favorite basic models. Here are examples of more complex models:

- Flipper by Enhanced Vision is a camera suspended in a hinged frame so it swings or "flips" 180 degrees. It is the only device that allows you to see your face or your art project, for example, on your TV screen, as well as reading material. Flipper can also be attached to glasses with a built-in screen, named Flipperport.

- Jordy by Enhanced Vision is a combination telescope, magnifier, and video camera. For distance viewing you wear it on your eyes, like a small pair of binoculars that automatically focuses at different distances. For reading you hang it on its holder and plug it into your TV. Since it has multiple capabilities, it is the most expensive of the tools in this section. Some people like it, others do not, so be sure to try it out before you purchase it.

MAGNIFIER TROUBLESHOOTING: WHAT HAPPENS IF YOUR BACK OR NECK FEELS STRAINED

If you're using a stand magnifier, you'll need a reading stand or adjustable table. Try to position the material and magnifier so they are high enough that your back can remain straight while you read. If you plan to read for a long time, create a special reading area in your home with a correctly adjusted table and chair that are comfortable for you. You can combine a reading stand that tilts the material to a comfortable angle with an adjustable-height table. You may also use the table for a CCTV. Some low-vision catalogs carry stands and tables, or you can purchase them at an office supply shop or a medical supply store. As unappealing as this may sound, hospital-type bed tables actually make great CCTV stands; they are adjustable, mobile, and strong.

Six Common Magnifier Mistakes

Mistake 1. Any Magnifier Will Work

It is very difficult for fully sighted people to understand that all magnifiers are not created equally. If you have full sight, it *is* true that any magnifier will work for you. Everything will look clear; it will just look a little bigger or a lot bigger, depending on the strength of the magnifier. But if you have macular degeneration, a magnifier that is not strong enough for you will not make everything look clear. Everything will still appear blurry. It won't work. That's why it's so important to buy magnifiers for close viewing in the right power (see "What Is My Diopter Power or X Power?" earlier).

Mistake 2. Bigger Magnifiers Make Things Bigger

The laws of physics dictate that the more powerful the magnifier, the smaller its lens. So bigger magnifiers are also weaker magnifiers. They cover a bigger area, but they don't make things that much bigger. If you find a huge hand-held magnifier in a store or catalog, or a magnifier that enlarges a whole page, you can bet that it's not more than a 2X, which means it will only make print appear two times its original size. If you need more magnification than that, you will need a smaller magnifier. With a smaller magnifier you will see more clearly, but you will see less print at a time (this is one of the reasons that many people who need strong magnifiers prefer CCTVs—they enable you to see more print at one time even though they magnify powerfully).

Mistake 3. Stronger Magnifiers Are Better

Do not buy the strongest magnifier on the market. Instead, buy the weakest magnifier you can use without straining. Why? Because the stronger the magnifier, the smaller its lens and the less area you will be able to see with it. For example, with a 2X magnifier you will be able to see the entire line on the next page. With a 5X magnifier you will see only the first four words. And holding a 7X magnifier, you will only see the first two words before you have to move the magnifier or the page. It's obviously much easier to read if you can see more words at a time, so you need to opt for the weakest magnifiers you can use without straining.

I can do this, especially if it's sunny. (2X)

I can do this. (5X)

I can. (7X)

Mistake 4. I Can Hold My Magnifier Any Which Way

This is probably the trickiest truth about magnifiers: you can't hold a magnifier at just any distance from an object and have it work. Sure, if you have one of those huge Sherlock Holmes magnifiers and you've got 20/20 vision you can hold it anywhere you'd like and it will work. But Sherlock Holmes's magnifier was pretty weak. We know that because it's very large and the larger the magnifier, the weaker it is. The minute you start using smaller, more powerful magnifiers, especially if you have low vision, you need to hold them at precisely the right distance from the object or print you want to see. Otherwise everything will look blurry. And if you move the magnifier back and forth, and up and down, you'll make yourself dizzy and nauseous.

So how do you know where to hold it? Place the magnifier on the object or print you want to see and then pull it up slowly until the object or print comes into focus. That is the correct distance from the object or print at which to hold the magnifier. This distance will never change for this particular magnifier. You can cement your hand to exactly that spot.

However, now you're only halfway done. You still have to figure out how far away from the magnifier your eye should be. Why does it make a difference where your eye is if the magnifier is already focused on the object or print you want to see? It makes a difference for the same reason that it makes a difference where you stand if you're trying to see into the neighbor's yard through a hole in your fence. If you stand several feet back from the hole, all you perceive is a tiny glimpse of green lawn on the other side. If you walk right up to the fence and look through the hole, though, you'll be able to see quite a large area of the neighbor's yard. A powerful magnifier works the same way. It is relatively small, like a little hole in a fence, so the farther away you hold your eye from its lens, the less you're going to see of the object or print you're looking at. Sure, whatever you see you'll see clearly, because you've focused the lens properly, but you will just see quite a small piece of it clearly.

If you want to see more of the object or print you're looking at with your magnifier, *keep the magnifier at the correct distance from the object or print and move BOTH the magnifier and the object together toward your eye. Alternatively, hold the magnifier right up to your eye and move the object close enough to bring it into focus.*

As you'll discover, the stronger the magnifier, the closer your eye will have to be to it, because it's essentially like a smaller hole in the fence. This is another reason that CCTVs are so popular. With a CCTV you can get very powerful magnification and still sit at a comfortable distance away from the screen. You can't do that with a magnifier. Because very high-powered reading glasses or magnifiers require such close handling and are sometimes tricky to select and use, your best bet is to have them professionally fitted by an eye doctor who specializes in low vision (see appendix A for contact information for offices in your area).

Mistake 5. Lighting Doesn't Matter

You need good light to see with a magnifier. Magnifiers have solid frames or edges that block light, and your hand, head, or shoulder can block light or cast shadows, especially when you hold material very close to your eyes. When you are evaluating magnifiers, make sure you have bright light directed onto the page. A regular shade lamp with an incandescent lightbulb is almost never a good-enough source of light. The bulb disperses the light into the room instead of onto the page, and the shade makes things even worse by muting much of the light, sending the remainder up to the ceiling and down to the floor. A gooseneck or flexible-arm lamp with an indoor floodlight bulb is much better. If glare is a problem, adjust the lamp so light shines from the side onto the page or consider using a lighted magnifier or magnifier mounted on a lamp. If you plan to use your magnifier in public or poorly lit areas where you do not control the light source, I recommend a lighted magnifier or a lightweight pocket flashlight or penlight. If you feel your magnifier isn't working, always check your lighting first.

Mistake 6. One Tool Should Do It All for Everyone

All of the tools in this chapter work, but they don't all work for all people or for all tasks. It's essential to understand that virtually no tool will allow you to see *both* near and far, like your bifocals do (actually, your bifocals can do this only because they are two tools in one—they have two different types of lenses blended together). You must have a complete toolbox of magnifiers and telescopes if you are going to see and do everything you want to see and do. Which ones you choose depend on a number of factors, including what power you need, your activities, your personal preferences, and, of course, your personal budget. Whatever you do, though, don't try to get one tool to do it all and then give up in frustration. No tool is designed to do it all.

TELESCOPES:
YOUR DISTANCE-VIEWING TOOLBOX

Telescopes work like binoculars. They help us see distant objects clearly by making them appear larger. You may have used one pair of binoculars for years to see all different kinds of things from birds in trees to football players on a field, just like you may have had one pair of bifocals to see everything nearby. But just as one magnifier won't meet all your needs, one telescope may not, either. The best telescope for a task depends on the task itself, whether you need both hands free, whether you need portability, how wide a field of view you need, how much area you need to see through the lens, and how much strength you need in the lens.

Get a Wide-Enough Field of View

Telescopes limit the width of your field of view, giving you the impression that you are looking at the world through a tunnel. In general, a telescope that gives you less than ten degrees of field is not very useful. Catalogs will usually list the field-of-view degrees for each telescope, but if they don't you should ask.

Power Is Different with Telescopes

Just so things wouldn't be too easy, it turns out that power works differently with telescopes than it does with magnifiers. With magnifiers, it's crucial to purchase one with the right X power or diopter for your level of vision. This rule is not as important with telescopes, because you're looking at something farther away, so the focus distance is more flexible. If you have pretty good vision, you can probably use a 2X or 2.8X. If you have very low vision, you will probably need something stronger, although there is no way to tell precisely without trying each telescope out.

When you look at telescopes listed in catalogs, you may notice that the lens strength is noted differently than it is with magnifiers. Instead of 4X, 8X, and so forth, you'll see telescopes listed in catalogs as 4X12 or 8X16 and so forth. The first number still indicates the X power of the lens (see "Diopters and X Powers" earlier). The second number indicates the diameter of the outer lens of the telescope. Why do we even need to know that? Well, the power divided into the diameter tells you the area in millimeters that you have to look through to use the telescope (not the breadth of your field of view). The larger that area is, the easier it will be to see through it. So a 4X12 telescope has $12/4=3$ millimeters of viewing area. An 8X16 has $16/8=$only 2 millimeters of viewing area. How much viewing area do you need? That depends on your unique pattern of vision: the size and location of the blind spots or scotomas on your macula (see chapter 11), your contrast sensitivity, and personal preference.

Telescopes for Stationary Viewing

These telescopes look like little binoculars mounted on an eyeglass frame. They're called binocular spectacles, television glasses, or sports spectacles in catalogs. You can use them to watch TV, the opera, a recital, or a sports event. Since they sit comfortably on your nose, you can watch something for a long time without wearing out your arm as you would if you were holding up a regular pair of binoculars. There are several good models. Lightweight 2X to 2.8X models are very popular and relatively inexpensive. Some people prefer clip-on monocular telescopes, which fit over one lens of your glasses.

Telescopes for Moving Around

If you already have a pair of binoculars, experiment with them first. Take them when you leave home and try reading street signs or store signs or seeing your bowling pins. If it works, but they are too heavy, consider the following:

- A lightweight pair of binoculars from a camping or sporting store or opera glasses.

- A handheld monocular telescope, to hold up to one eye. This will easily fit in a pocket or purse or can hang around your neck on its own cord. Some models can be attached to small handles. The 4X12 with variable focus gives a relatively strong power, a wide field, and a range of distances. Monoculars are a little harder to get used to using than binoculars but have the advantage of less weight and bulk. My father has used one for bowling for years.

- Custom-made bioptic lenses, which are small telescopes mounted in an eyeglass frame, or special telescopes like the VES and VesMini by Designs for Vision. Some people can also use these types of lenses for driving (see chapter 13). You must purchase these from a low-vision optometrist or ophthalmologist or a rehabilitation program. They are among the most expensive products listed in this chapter.

Multipurpose Telescopes: For Seeing Far and Near

The Jordy by Enhanced Vision is both an auto-focus telescope and a video camera that plugs into your TV and turns it into a CCTV. It also appears in the section on CCTVs. The Beecher Mirage is a variable-focus telescope that has a snap-on lens cap for near viewing.

COMPUTERS AND SOFTWARE: FOR YOUR ELECTRONIC TOOLBOX

If you already own a computer, you may be surprised to discover how much it can do for you. If you don't own one but wish you did, this might be the best time of all to buy. Like magnifiers, computers are fabulous tools for people with vision loss. They're now sold with large monitors that feature adjustable brightness and color for better contrast with less glare. You can also change the font sizes on your screen to read more easily.

With special software, your computer can read your e-mail or any of its files aloud to you in a nice voice, and it can follow voiced instructions that you give it. You can also buy a scanner that will read any typed page out loud and then transmit it to your computer. All it takes is the right hardware, the right software, and the determination to tackle a learning curve in order to get the hang of it.

There are many excellent products out on the market, but most of my patients who use computers find the first three of the following software options to be the most helpful. See appendix C for the contact information for all of the companies mentioned here. Software is developing so rapidly that we have not given specific versions or prices. Contact the manufacturers or computer retailers listed in appendix C for the latest versions available and pricing.

Accessibility Features Already Built into Your Computer

These features are already built into most computers, although we're often not aware that they're there. Basic accessibility features allow you to enlarge the print on your screen and to vary the background and print colors to achieve maximum contrast with minimum glare. For example, you can flip the colors of your print so that you read bright white letters on a dark black screen. For many folks, these features alone make it much easier to read E-mail and type documents. Some newer computers also include built-in "voice input," which means the computer will follow verbal directions as well as keyboard directions. You can usually find the accessibility features on your computer by clicking on either "My Computer" or "Help" or "Support."

GOOD ADVICE

Be sure to check the system requirements for software before you purchase it. They are printed on the outside of the software packaging or in the product description section of the catalog. If you cannot find the system requirements, insist on talking to a sales representative to make sure that you understand them before you purchase your software. Most software is not returnable, especially once it has been opened.

"System requirements" are the minimum qualities that a software program requires your computer to have in order to run smoothly. They usually include a certain amount of memory or RAM, a certain amount of space on your hard drive, a certain-speed processor, and an operating system compatible with the software program. If your computer is more than four years old or not very powerful, you may have to purchase additional RAM, a faster processor, or a larger hard drive or even upgrade to a new computer in order to use some of the software programs featured in this chapter.

Print Enlargement Programs

You can use screen enlargement software on any computer and with any size monitor, but the larger the monitor, the easier it will be to see more words on the screen at a time. Screen enlargement software magnifies the words on the screen up to 16 or 20x. That means the print will be sixteen to twenty times larger than regular-sized print, which is enough magnification so that most people with macular degeneration can read anything on the screen. There are at least six different screen enlargement software programs on the market, but my patients find the most success with these two: ZoomText Level 1 by AiSquared and MAGic by Henter-Joyce, which may have an easier menu.

Combo Print Enlargement and Talking Computer Programs

With this software, your computer can enlarge its print or read to you whatever appears on its screen, or it can do both at the same time. If you have hearing impairments or find it difficult to hear soft or stilted voices, you may find the computer's speech hard to understand, although you can still use the print enlargement features. This software also provides shortcut keys that make navigating around to different commands or pages easier. As with regular screen enlargement software, my patients find the most success with these two brands: ZoomText by AiSquared and MAGic by Henter-Joyce, which may have better speech quality.

Talking Computer Programs

These powerful programs read aloud, but they do not enlarge print. They are most useful for people with severe visual impairments who do not read even very large print. If you have a hearing impairment or find it difficult to hear soft or stilted voices, you may not be able to hear the computer's voice clearly enough to use these programs. My patients and colleagues find the most success with these two brands: JAWS for Windows by Freedom Scientific and Window-Eyes by G. W. Micro, which may be easier to use than JAWS.

Voice Recognition Programs

If you find using a computer keyboard difficult, you can purchase voice recognition software that allows your computer to recognize your voice and follow your spoken instructions. It can even take dictation, typing up on your screen whatever you say out loud. My patients and colleagues find the following three programs to be the best: L&H Voice Xpress by Lernout & Hauspie, ViaVoice by IBM, and Dragon Naturally Speaking by Dragon Systems.

NEED COMPUTER TUTORING?

If you are considering more complex
software programs, contact your local
rehabilitation program and your State
Commission for the Blind and ask
them about free or low-cost computer
training for the visually impaired. If
you have veterans' benefits, the VA
offers these classes in some selected
locations. Just between you and me,
though, sometimes these classes are
designed for young people with vision
loss and may use teaching styles that
assume you can easily follow computer
commands and remember them with
little review. You may have a
wonderful experience. But if you don't
succeed in a particular class, don't be
discouraged or take it personally. It's
not a reflection of your ability to learn
computers and software.

Reading Scanners and Braille Computers

Reading scanners and Braille computers are very
popular in the blind community, but they can

also be very effective for people with low vision who find scanners useful or who decide to learn Braille. As with the more complex software programs, these hardware options require training to use easily. If you decide to purchase a reading scanner, make sure it is compatible with your computer.

Scanners, as the name suggests, can scan any typewritten text onto your computer screen as a text file. Kurzweil and AiSquared offer scanners, but one that deserves special mention is Arkenstone's OPENbook, which combines scanning with voice output, essentially turning your computer into a scanning and talking reading machine.

Braille computers translate whatever appears on your computer screen into Braille, and you can also type in Braille. Portable note takers, the Braille version of a laptop notebook, can print out in Braille and read aloud. The leading companies for these machines are Blazie Engineering and Pulse Data/HumanWare. Prices vary greatly.

Voice-Activated PDAs

Voice-activated PDAs (Personal Desk Assistants) are the Palm Pilots of low vision. They can do just about everything a regular PDA can do, but better because you don't need to see to use them. They feature voice input, output, voice notepad and dictaphone, talking calculator and currency converter, voiced appointment book, and meeting planner, and they upload to your PC just like a regular PDA. The most popular brand is Parrot's Voice Mate.

Getting Computer Advice from the People Who Know

Sometimes the best people to ask for computer advice are not the experts but the folks like you who have been there themselves and discovered the lay of the land the hard way. They understand what you'll find most difficult or most helpful. To ask questions or find answers from others with low vision, go to Screen Magnifier's Web site at www.magnifiers.org. Screen Magnifiers is an independent nonprofit organization that provides free information about software and hardware products and the Internet for people with vision loss. You can view archived reviews and articles on their site or sign up for their E-mail group to ask specific questions. You can also join the on-line community MD Support at www.mdsupport.org, where you'll find lots of information. Join their E-mail group to ask specific questions and get lots of good war stories about computers and software.

CHAPTER 13

Saving Sight on the Road: Driving, Alternatives, and Traveling

When I lost my license I thought, you might as well shoot me. Why do I want to live if I can't drive?
—John Patrick Reynolds

I first met Celia when she agreed to drive for me. Now she's become one of my very best friends. What a funny way life has of giving you gifts when you least expect them.
—Bixley Bennett

For just about everyone, except perhaps for folks in New York City who've never owned cars, losing one's license may be the worst blow that macular degeneration delivers. I have heard many people, like Pat Reynolds, tell me that they'd rather not live than not drive. We've grown to accept cars as essential to our lifestyle, but they are more than just vehicles for getting around. We see them as representations of our personal style, success, sense of security, and even sexuality. They are part of our memories. Remember the beautiful twelve-cylinder Lincoln Zephyrs and the smart Studebakers parading down the avenues after World War II? Remember your first car? Your favorite car?

The great irony of our love affair with cars is that they don't necessarily love us back. They're expensive, they encourage us to be dependent on them, they contribute to pollution that causes global warming, they divert funds from public transportation, and they require that we see well enough to pass our state's license exam. That's not what I call a supportive relationship.

Every time I talk to people who have just returned from a trip to some great European city like Paris or Munich, they rave about how wonderful the public transportation is there and how nice it is to get around town without driving. Each time I think, What are we doing? Shouldn't we be just as committed to public transportation here—just as willing to use it and just as vocal to our legislators about its value? Wouldn't it be nice to see ourselves independently of our cars? Well, we can—we must, really—because otherwise we will just drive ourselves nuts and wind up inside the house every day. That's no way to live.

The good news is that there are lots of alternatives to cars. We just have to seek them out and start using them. In the meantime, if your vision loss is mild you may still be eligible to drive. This chapter explains all of your options.

YOUR LICENSE AND THE DEPARTMENT OF MOTOR VEHICLES (DMV)

As you know, vision test results on a 20/20 scale are the Holy Grail of the DMV. They take these test scores as the gospel truth about whether or not you're able to drive safely, which is puzzling, since the research on driving just doesn't support that conclusion. The 20/20 scale measures only visual acuity (how crisply you see static printed letters on a chart or screen). It doesn't measure other factors that directly contribute to driving competence, like contrast sensitivity (whether you can distinguish objects from a similarly colored background), dynamic acuity (how well you see when you're actually driving rather than when you're standing motionless in the DMV), glare sensitivity, processing time (how quickly your mind synthesizes visual information), reaction time (how quickly you react physically when you realize what's happening), or a sense of one's own mortality. The most dangerous drivers on the road today are not people with mild low vision from macular degeneration but young men under twenty-five with excellent vision and terrible judgment.

339

A movement is underway among low vision professionals to change the state DMV driving requirements to better reflect current research, but until that happens we all have to live with the current rules, which are more complex than you might think. Each state has its own vision requirements for driving, and no two are alike (Canadian readers see appendix F).

Driving with Visual Aids

More than half the states allow drivers to use special bioptic telescopes for driving. These tiny telescopes are mounted on your regular eyeglass frame and used for seeing stoplights and traffic signs. Many people with the juvenile form of macular degeneration, called Stargardt's disease, drive successfully with these telescopes. These optical aids are also available to people with age-related macular degeneration, although a couple of catches make them less appealing for older people than they are for younger adults.

First, bioptic telescopes must be prescribed by an ophthalmologist or optometrist and are usually quite expensive, costing between $500 and $1,000. The state may also require that you pay for a special driver training class. Then you must pass the driving test, with the likelihood of no refund for either the telescopes or the training should you not pass. Medicare does not cover bioptic telescopes for driving, and private insurance rarely covers them.

Second, age-related macular degeneration often does more extensive damage to the retina than Stargardt's disease does. With AMD, you may not be able to use bioptic telescopes as effectively as someone with Stargardt's can. AMD is also progressive, so you may be able to use your bioptic telescopes for only a relatively short period of time before you lose additional vision. However, some people do keep a significant amount of vision with macular degeneration for many years.

If you would like to try bioptic telescopes, check with your DMV office to see if they are permissible and contact your doctor for a referral to a low-vision ophthalmologist or optometrist or visit a visual rehabilitation program. You may also want to read Eli and Doron Peli's book *Driving with Confidence: A Practical Guide to Driving with Low Vision*, which is printed in large type, and contact a low-vision driver training specialist in your area who is familiar with your state's test. See appendix D for contact information.

Driving with a Restricted License

If you have less than the required vision in either one or both eyes (20/40 in most states), you may qualify for a restricted license that allows you to drive under limited conditions, such as only during daylight, in your neighborhood, or under a certain speed limit. The vision minimums for a restricted license vary widely. For example, as of 2002 New York's minimum was 20/70, North Carolina's was 20/100, and California's was 20/200. Contact your local DMV office or visit your state's DMV Web site for current restricted license information. Remember, if your doctor writes a letter endorsing your ability to drive, he or she must also state that you have vision that meets the state's requirements on a 20/20 scale; otherwise, you will be denied a license regardless of what else your doctor may say about your capabilities.

Tips for Taking the DMV Tests

- **Know The Whole Story Before You Go**
  In many states, you only need good vision in one eye to qualify for a license. However, the clerk may mistakenly deny your application or comment on your limited vision. Don't be intimidated. Know your state's DMV rules before you go for testing and mention them if necessary. Find out ahead of time if you are eligible for a restricted license and request one if necessary. If your DMV office has poor lighting or you suspect that the vision-

testing machine may underestimate your vision, call ahead and ask if you can be evaluated at your doctor's office. Many states allow you to use these results instead, but they will not be valid once you take the DMV's test.

- **Put Your Best Foot Forward**
Consider practicing driving on the streets in the vicinity of the DMV ahead of time so that you are familiar with the area, the lights, and the traffic patterns. Practice at the same time of day that you will be taking your driving test. Go for testing on a good-weather day when you feel rested and focused. Do not go at dusk or when it's raining. Dress in your nicest or most businesslike outfit. Square your shoulders and walk in with confidence. Keep in mind that you may be observed from the moment you enter the building for signs of alert awareness and competence. During the driving test, wear amber-colored sunglasses or lenses to reduce glare and increase your contrast perception.

- **Remember That the First Word Isn't Final**
Do not accept the decision of any single DMV employee on your ability to drive according to the state's regulations. If you

are rejected, keep calm and request a full reevaluation.

Should I Keep Driving?

Of course, the law dictates that you may not drive if your vision is below the minimum required for licensure in your state, even if your state's vision requirements are arbitrary and do not actually reflect your ability to drive safely (as unfair as this is). Since driving is central to daily life for most Americans and our vision is tested infrequently, especially by the DMV, many people with macular degeneration still have valid licenses, would like to continue driving, and wonder when they should make the decision to stop.

Some folks with macular degeneration still have good acuity, but since acuity is only one factor among many that makes a driver safe, they sometimes sense that they nevertheless aren't as effective on the road as they'd like to be. "I stopped driving even though my doctor said I could still see well enough," Dolly Kowalski told me, "because I said to myself, What if I hit a child? I couldn't live with that." Dolly's decision turned out to be wise given her particular pattern of vision. She has very low contrast sensitivity, which makes it difficult for her to see objects against similarly colored backgrounds. Darting children in cream-colored jackets playing by tan-colored cars on a light gray concrete street would be hard for her to see, even though her acuity is technically quite good. Other folks drive until they have a surprising near miss or a minor accident—a brush with a parked car or a collision with the garage door frame. Yet others continue to drive quite safely while their vision is still strong. So what should you do?

If you have any doubts, do not drive. If you are unsure about the quality of your vision, you can ask your low-vision optometrist or ophthalmologist or visual rehabilitation program to assess your vision and talk with you about driving (see appendix A for contact information). You might also want to consider the following questions, which were inspired by Eli and Doron Peli's self-test in *Driving with Confidence: A Practical Guide to Driving with Low Vision.*

The Macular Degeneration Driving Self-Test

1. When you are driving, do objects like other cars or pedestrians catch you by surprise? Do they seem to appear out of nowhere?

2. Have you recently not seen another car until the driver honked or not seen a parked vehicle until you were right next to it? Do other drivers honk at you for no apparent reason?

3. Do you have a stiff neck or limited neck rotation? Do you find it difficult to turn your

head and scan the whole landscape in front of you?

4. Have you noticed that your reflexes are much slower than they used to be and your reaction time is much longer? Does it take you a number of seconds to react to an event on the road?

5. Do you ever feel momentarily confused or unsure when you are driving? Does driving make you nervous or uncomfortable?

6. Has a family member or friend suggested that you stop driving and given you examples of why he or she thinks so?

7. Do you have low contrast sensitivity? Do you find it relatively difficult to distinguish an object that is sitting against a background of the same color?

8. Is your visual acuity on a 20/20 scale below the minimum level required by your state?

Pearls of Wisdom for Driving

If you answered "no" to the self-test questions above, then you can feel confident continuing to drive. You may want to follow these pearls:

- **Start Using Alternatives Today**
  Use public transportation and other alternatives as much as you can while you have your license. This may feel like giving up some precious driving time too early, but it's very savvy. Better to feel confident and in control of the future than to let it catch you by surprise.

- **Take an AARP 55 Alive Course**
  This course offers a special curriculum for drivers over fifty-five to sharpen their general driving skills. See appendix D for classes in your area.

- **Drive Strategically**
  Plan ahead to avoid driving at the riskiest times: at dusk, when it's more difficult to see, and when you are rushed or tired.

- **Wear Glare-Blocking Sunglasses**
  Wear amber-colored sunglasses or lenses to reduce glare from sunlight and snow and increase your contrast perception (see the catalog listings in appendix C).

- **Share a Ride**
  Consider calling a friend who doesn't drive and offering to share a ride. We're all in this crazy adventure called life together.

What better way to enjoy it than sharing the road?

WHEN DRIVING IS NO LONGER POSSIBLE

If you answered "yes" to any of the preceding self-test questions, then you probably should not continue to drive before consulting your doctor, especially at dusk or at night, at high speeds, or on busy streets. If you answered yes to number 8, then you definitely should not be driving. But do not despair. You are not the sum total of your car, and neither is your life. Keep reading! There are many other options for getting around town, traveling, and being active and engaged with friends, family, and the world.

Hooray for Alternatives!

As you know better than anyone, it's very difficult to give up driving (see chapter 6); but a number of alternatives can enable you to remain independent and continue doing the things that you enjoy. If you are thinking of moving, consider living within an easy distance of the places you'd like to go and factoring alternative modes of transportation into your decision on where to relocate.

Walking

Walking is incredibly beneficial for your health. Many of the healthiest seniors I've met walk between one half mile and three miles a day. They walk to the store, the post office, and the park, to volunteer at organizations and neighbors' homes, and just for pleasure or exercise. Walking is a particularly good option if you have strong bones and good balance. Plan your routes to cross at lighted crosswalks. Consider carrying lightweight binoculars or a monocular telescope to read traffic lights and street signs and to see storefronts and people at a distance. Wear amber-colored sunglasses (see appendix C) to reduce glare and increase contrast sensitivity, which makes seeing irregularities in the sidewalk easier. I also recommend carrying a lightweight collapsible white identification cane (see chapter 14), which you can use when crossing busy streets to alert drivers and induce them to be more careful.

Riding Three-Wheeled Bikes and Battery-Powered Scooters

While walking has tremendous benefits, it often precludes carrying packages or purchases, especially if they're heavy. For bringing goods home, try taking a lightweight wheeled shopping cart with you or riding a three-wheeled bike with a large basket or a battery-powered scooter, especially if the sidewalks are good in your area. Unlike golf carts, battery-powered scooters are only as wide as a person and go at walking speed. You can also ride your three-wheel bike at walking speed. Use the tips from "Walking" earlier and remember to be especially cautious when crossing streets, since you may be riding below the level of some drivers' line of vision. Some people put a bicycle flag on their bike or scooter for greater visibility.

Shopping carts are inexpensive and available at your local mart. Bikes and battery-powered scooters vary in price. Call your local bike retailer to ask about three-wheeled bikes and see appendix C for scooter manufacturer information. If you are a veteran, you may be eligible for a free or subsidized battery-powered scooter. Contact your local VA office or call 800-827-1000 for information.

Hiring and Sharing Drivers

If you sell your car and take all the money you once spent on it—in gas, insurance, and maintenance—you probably can afford to hire a driver with a car at least once a week. If you were to pool your money with a friend or two who live nearby, you could hire a driver for several days a week. There may be high school seniors, college students, community volunteers, or even family members who would welcome the opportunity to drive for you part-time. Alternatively, you could arrange to loan your own car indefinitely to a family member or trusted friend with the clear agreement that he or she pay for the extra gas used and be your driver a few times a week. Remember, outside of the convenience, there's nothing inherently special about driving yourself around; the richest people in the world have chauffeurs.

Taking Taxis

If you live in a city with many taxis and many competitive customers, consider carrying a neon yellow card at least five by eight inches high with the word TAXI written in large black print. Hold the card up when you need a ride, and a taxi will find you. You can make a card yourself or order one from a low-vision catalog.

If you live in a metropolitan area with fewer taxis and you have friends with low vision, consider scheduling a regular weekly or biweekly shared taxi ride to lunch, the hairstylist, shopping centers, or religious services. Taxi companies in low-traffic areas tend to be more responsive to regular or prescheduled customers than to last-minute calls. However, they are not always prompt. Build in a certain amount of additional time so that you aren't rushed.

Using Senior Transit and Para-Transit

Many public transportation departments offer special transportation services for seniors, as do some churches, mosques, synagogues, senior centers, and community centers. Check with your clergy, county, or city offices for more information. Usually these services provide door-to-door transportation in a small bus or van to doctors' offices and other select locations, although some transit programs will take you anywhere you'd like to go in the area. You may need to make reservations and have patience, but the service may be free or cost less than public transportation.

Riding Buses, Subways, and Light Rail

Learning to use public transportation can take a few trips and lots of courage, but once you've learned it, it's relatively easy. In cities like New York, where many people with perfect vision don't own cars and places are closer together, public transportation is actually the best way to travel and you can do it with low vision, too. To familiarize yourself with the bus system in your area and to become confident using it, try the following four steps.

FOUR STEPS TO RIDING THE BUS

1. Call your public transportation authority for maps and schedules. If the print is too small, enlarge it on a photocopy machine. Many transportation authorities offer specific route information by phone for the visually impaired. Ask about discount fares for seniors or the disabled and prepurchased passes. You may also want to ask for a bus mitten, which looks like an oven mitt embossed with the transportation authority's logo. You can hold it up to signal the bus driver to stop. If there is no bus mitten for your area, you can make a large-print sign that says: "BUS: PLEASE STOP" and hold it up when you suspect the bus may be coming.

2. If you plan to pay with coins, count out your bus fare at home and put it in a separate pocket so that it's easily available. Hold a white identification cane at the bus stop or tell the driver that you have low vision. Ask whether you are boarding the right bus. Drivers are often required to assist riders by announcing stops by name and will be especially helpful if they know you have low vision. Request a seat at the very front of the bus so that you can hear the driver and he or she doesn't forget you. The law requires that these seats be given to people with disabilities.

3. The first time you use the bus, go with a friend or family member and have him or her show you how to do it. The second time, have your friend or family member simply tag along; make all the decisions yourself. Practice this way until you are completely comfortable with the routine. Once you have no difficulties, you're ready to use the bus alone.

4. Although mishaps are unlikely, have a contingency plan in case you miss your stop or the bus is very late. Your plan may include knowing the routes fairly well, bringing extra fare or taxi fare, and carrying change for a pay phone and a friend's or family member's phone number or a preprogrammed voice-activated cell phone. Keep an ear to the weather report, too. On very cold or very hot days, you might want to opt for another alternative if the bus service in your area is not reliable.

THE FOUR STEPS FOR RIDING SUBWAYS AND LIGHT RAIL

You can use steps 1, 3, and 4 for the subway and light rail, too. With subways and light rail, it's also important to figure out where the train cars usually stop on the platform, so you can anticipate where the doors will be before they open.

Double-check with other passengers that you're boarding the right car and count the stops in your head or with your fingers so that you know when to disembark. Buy tokens or subway tickets in bulk so that you don't have to fiddle with the fare machines every time you go.

TRAVELING AWAY FROM HOME

"I used to go to Hawaii every February to visit my brother," Caroline Smedley told me one day in my office, "but I don't think I'll go now."

"But why not?" I said.

"Well," she sighed, "I just think it would be too hard with my vision loss."

She's right, it probably will be hard, especially the first time she travels. But it's not impossible, it gets easier, and there couldn't be a more important thing Caroline could possibly do than enjoy a vacation with her brother in Hawaii. Vision loss is hard enough as it is. Why make it harder by depriving yourself of something you really enjoy?

Caroline was probably thinking of a million little worries that added up in her mind: How will I change planes in Los Angeles? How will I be able to set up my things in an unfamiliar bathroom? What if everyone wants to watch a movie or play cards and I can't see either? These are all natural worries, but are they really valid?

For almost every concern there's an answer. After all, blind adults have been traveling and visiting friends for decades, and the people who care about you want to see you regardless of your vision. And you can still see a great deal of the world even with macular degeneration. The trick is not to get caught up in how you've always done things but look for new ways to make the world accessible for you.

Tips

- **The Early Bird Gets the Worm**
  Travel is so much less stressful if you leave yourself enough room to make mistakes and enough time to relax.

- **Keep Key Information at Your Fingertips**
  Write important information like flight numbers, phone numbers, and medications in large print with a black felt-tip pen so you can read it easily, or carry a pocket tape recorder and tape it all for easy playback. Alternatively, carry a preprogrammed voice-activated cell phone or a calling card number and a voice-activated personal desk assistant (called a PDA or "palm pilot" after the popular brand). See the low-vision catalogs in appendix C for PDAs.

- **Pack for Maximum Ease**
  Pack neutral-color clothes or clothes in
  the same color family for easy matching;
  use separate plastic bags or tags for
  matching outfits. Use brightly colored
  cosmetic bags to organize items in your
  purse and suitcase so they're easier to
  find. Put brightly colored, contrasting
  tape on both sides of your luggage so
  it's easily identifiable. Purchase or
  make yourself large-print luggage
  tags with black block lettering that's
  easy to read.

- **Keep Your Money Handy**
  Carry a small roll of new one-dollar bills
  for easy tipping. Organize your money
  using the tips in chapter 14. Be cautious
  with your purse or briefcase, but do not
  fear. Research shows that people with low
  vision are not at greater risk for crime in
  otherwise safe places, such as U.S. and
  Canadian airports.

- **Make Travel Entertaining**
  Take a handheld four-track or regular tape
  player or a CD player and a selection of
  taped books, magazines, and music with
  you. Bring your large-print playing cards,
  crossword puzzles, and any other games
  you enjoy.

- **Adapt the New Location to You**
  Bring your own alarm clock with big
  buttons and a desktop gooseneck lamp
  with an indoor floodlight bulb if you often
  use one. Spend time familiarizing yourself
  with your hotel room or your friend's
  home. Arrange your belongings for
  maximum visibility. You can even call
  ahead of time, ask about the facilities, and
  pack whatever you think might be helpful,
  including contrasting-color towels for the
  bathroom.

- **The Squeaky Wheel Gets the Grease**
  As you know all too well, most people with
  full vision have no idea what it's like to
  live with low vision. They probably won't
  be able to guess your needs or your
  feelings. In fact, half the time they won't
  realize what you can and can't see—or
  they'll make the wrong assumption. So the
  best solution is to speak up—ask for what
  you want and you will probably get it. Ask
  the flight attendant to show you to the
  bathroom; ask the waiter to list the
  entrées if the restaurant doesn't have a
  big-print menu; ask your friends to turn up
  the lights and play with your cards rather
  than theirs. Explain your vision when you
  need to. Do the best you can to make the

world work for you—and have patience when it doesn't. All the best things in life take effort, and all the best relationships require compromise.

Flying on Airplanes

- **Prearrange Assistance**
Federal law now mandates that people with low vision have equal access when traveling. If you give the airline at least forty-eight hours' notice, they must assist you in changing planes. This may involve accepting a wheelchair ride from one gate to the other. I know that you may feel uncomfortable appearing in a wheelchair in public when you don't use one at home. But this is not the time to let pride thwart your travel plans. In a wheelchair you get a comfortable, stress-free ride while everyone else has to rush through the crowds. Who's the smarter one?

- **Let People Know You Have Low Vision**
If you arrive at the airport with a friend, tell the ticket counter clerk that you have low vision and request a pass so that your friend can accompany you to your gate. When you reach your gate, tell the staff you have low vision. They must allow you

to preboard or assist you with boarding and deplaning at your request (although they may ask you to wait until other passengers have disembarked first). Consider carrying a white identification cane or wearing a low-vision button (see chapter 14) in the airport even if you don't use one at home. It can work like magic. The airline is required by law to give you up-to-date information on your flight if you cannot read the monitors in the terminal. If you use a white cane, employees will know right away that they should answer your questions and other passengers will probably be much more receptive. Tell your flight attendant, too, so that he or she can be helpful.

• **Use Optical Aids**
Use your lighted handheld magnifier for reading tickets and your binoculars or monocular for seeing gate numbers. You can also take the same glasses for use on board as you use to watch your TV at home, although plane TV monitors are often difficult to see (even for the fully sighted).

• **Know Your Rights**
Although such occurrences are rare, if you feel you have been unfairly treated as a

result of having low vision you can request to speak with the airline's Complaints Resolution Official (CRO) or write to the airline directly. Mistreating good consumers is bad business, and airline management knows it. If you use a wheelchair, see appendix D for additional information on your rights.

- **Enjoy Your Flight**
  The sky might be a bit bumpy sometimes, but what a pleasure to spend time with folks you don't usually get to see or to visit someplace new. Enjoy it.

ADVENTURING FOR YEARS TO COME

As Helen Keller once said, "Life is a daring adventure or nothing at all." As she showed us throughout her life, there are lots of adventures to be had no matter who you are or how much you can see. There are many more things you can do in your home and around your community to make your life easier and more enjoyable. They're featured in our visual rehabilitation program here at Henry Ford Health System Eye Care Services in Michigan, and we've written them all down for you in the next chapter.

CHAPTER 14

Saving Sight at Home and in Your Community

I have a simple philosophy. Fill what's
empty. Empty what's full. And scratch
where it itches.
    —Alice Roosevelt Longworth

Who shall say I am not the happy
genius of my household?
    —William Carlos Williams

Give to the world the best you have,
and the best will come back to you.
    —Madeline Bridge

SAVING SIGHT AT HOME

Your home is your haven. There, at least, you can arrange your shelves the way you like them, put floodlights in the living room, and turn up the radio. This chapter will help you arrange your home for maximum visibility and ease. It begins with a few tips that will be helpful for the whole house and then looks at each room and makes more specific suggestions. For more detailed lighting and magnifier advice, please see Chapters 10 and 12. After we talk about your home, we'll head out into the community.

FOR EVERY ROOM IN YOUR HOME

Increasing Contrast and Decreasing Pattern

If you have macular degeneration, increasing contrast will make any object immediately more visible. Increasing contrast means increasing the color contrast or dark–light contrast between an object and its background. For example, a black pen on a white tablecloth has great contrast, while a black pen on a black tablecloth has no contrast. Objects that do not contrast with their backgrounds may disappear. A white saltshaker on a white tablecloth might as well be wearing camouflage in the jungle. The idea is to increase contrast wherever you can in your home. There are many ways to do so. For example, if certain doorways, furniture, or stairs are difficult to see, have them painted contrasting colors or use contrasting slipcovers or tablecloths. For hard-to-see glass coffee tables, put a brightly colored coffee table book on the edge of the table to make it more visible.

Decreasing pattern means decreasing color confusion (which is essentially another way to increase contrast). *Pattern* refers to multicolored designs or backgrounds. Flowered plates, bedsheets, and bank checks are examples of pattern. Pattern provides terrible contrast. Peas on a pretty flowered plate will be much harder to find than peas on a white plate. Similarly, a utensil or pen will be harder to find on a plaid tablecloth than on a plain contrasting one. While you're increasing contrast in your home, try to decrease pattern, too.

You can use contrast to redecorate your home for greater visibility without sacrificing style. Choose carpeting, furniture, fabrics, and wall paint in contrasting colors. For example, a cream carpet, forest green couch with cream print throw pillows, and mahogany coffee table is a much better choice than a cream carpet, beige couch, and glass coffee table.

Labeling and Organizing

Now you can use the labeling supplies you collected for this chapter (see chapter 9). Just about anything in your home can be labeled, including meters, switches, dials, buttons, clothing, clothing hangers, bottles, and boxed or canned goods. You don't have to label everything, though. Often you can use organizing instead of labeling to help you identify items quickly. For example, if you put chicken soup cans in one row, split-pea in a second row, and minestrone in a third, you don't have to label the cans to know which is which. You can also distinguish brown socks from blue ones by keeping them in separate drawers and washing them in separate netted hosiery bags. Labeling, however, can be especially valuable for hard-to-see dials and buttons or for things you absolutely don't want to mix up, such as prescription medications. When labeling, try to simplify by marking only the most frequently used settings or buttons (300 and 350 degrees on your stove, for example, the preferred room temperature on your thermostat, or the "permanent press" cycle setting on your washer).

Open Space

Don't save things. I know it's tempting, but it will cause you more headaches than it will spare. Extra jars, old files, and last year's clothing all create clutter and crowd closets and shelves. Blocked pathways and objects piled on steps are hazardous. Clearing as much open space as possible in your home will make everything easier to locate, it will make your home easier to clean, and it may be safer. As a rule, if you haven't used something or worn it for a year, it needs to go. If you are concerned about waste, recycle your containers and contribute your clothing to charity, but don't save.

Predictability

Predictability in your home is enormously important if you have macular degeneration. You can compensate for a lot of sight with predictability. The more predictable your home is, the better. You will always know where everything is. For small items that move around a lot, like house keys, wallets, and glasses, designate a spot for them and try to return them to that spot whenever you come home or put them aside. If you always do, you'll never have to spend an hour searching.

Finding Things

If you drop a pen on the floor or find yourself looking for a bottle of ketchup that could be anywhere in the refrigerator, scan systematically. To find the pen, sweep your hands along the floor from right to left or from your knees outward. To find the ketchup, begin searching at the top or bottom of the refrigerator and work your way from left to right on each shelf. If the ketchup bottle continues to disappear (which can happen if you are living with someone else), try labeling it with a rubber band so you will know it when you touch it, and assign it an agreed-upon location in the refrigerator.

Lighting and Magnifiers

Good glare-free lighting is essential for seeing just about anything in your home, and magnifiers are often helpful. See chapter 10 for advice on improving lighting and chapter 12 for advice on magnifiers and other visual aids. For detailed work or reading small print in any room, you may find a small gooseneck table lamp or a gooseneck floor lamp with an indoor floodlight bulb and a small lightweight flashlight helpful. You may also find a wide range of handheld and stand magnifiers, lighted magnifiers, and magnifying lamps very helpful.

PRODUCT SUGGESTIONS

Selected helpful products are highlighted in boxes in this chapter. These lists are not comprehensive. They are meant to suggest the wide range of products available through the low-vision catalogs listed in appendixes B and C. If you are hearing-impaired, you may need talking books and products with male voices, since female voices with higher pitches may be difficult to hear.

FOR YOUR LIVING ROOM

The rooms we spend the most time in, such as our living room, are often dimly lit or bathed in bright, glaring sunlight. Either extreme may make it very difficult for you to see well enough to enjoy watching television or using a magnifier to read. Adapt the light in these rooms with good lamps and sheer curtains or blinds. Reduce glare by covering shiny surfaces with tablecloths or heavy, secured area rugs or by wearing amber- or plum-tinted sunglasses (see chapter 10).

Television, Videos, and Radio

- Position your television away from reflecting or bright light, and *sit close to it*. If you still have trouble seeing the screen, try Coil focusable telescope glasses or a screen enlarger. Screen enlargers sit directly in front of your television, magnifying the whole screen by about 25 percent, although they also give you a narrow viewing angle.

- Use a giant-button remote. You can also mark the television buttons or dial with a contrasting permanent marker or puff paint.

- Try watching television shows or videos with Descriptive Video Service (see appendix B).

- Avoid local news broadcasts if you find their focus on crime stressful. Try national news programs instead.

- Radio is an excellent source of sports broadcasts, news, documentaries, concerts, variety shows, and religious programs. Try the National Public Radio (NPR) station in your area for a wide selection of programming.

Books, Magazines, and Newspapers

We often think of reading as the activity of looking at print on a page, but there are actually three different kinds of reading we can do: we can read visually, aurally, or tactilely. While we're most familiar with reading visually, that doesn't mean it's necessarily the best or the most enjoyable or the easiest way to read.

- Check out the amazing variety of free large-print and audiotaped newspapers, magazines, and books you can borrow or receive from the organizations listed in appendix B. Many favorites, such as *Newsweek*, *Discover*, *Reader's Digest*, and *US News and World Report*, are available. The National Library Service (NLS) has a wonderful program with new titles announced every month. NLS tapes must be played on a four-track player, which comes with your membership. You can also purchase your own four-track tape player from one of the low-vision catalogs listed in appendix C. Many local libraries also have extensive audiobook collections that use regular tape players.

- Choose from the thousands of large-print and audiotaped books for sale at your local bookstore, through on-line bookstores, or through the book clubs listed in appendix B.

- If you'd like to try reading in Braille, the Hadley School for the Blind offers free correspondence courses for people with low vision and their families (see appendix B for contact information). They're working on a new class using Jumbo Braille, which should be easy to learn. Braille is especially good for reading poetry and labeling items in your home.

TIPS FOR VISUAL READING

- If you read best with high-powered reading glasses, prop your elbows on the arms of the chair to comfortably maintain a close reading distance.

- Whenever you read, make sure adequate light shines directly on the page. Most people prefer a strong, adjustable gooseneck floor lamp or table lamp with an indoor flood-light bulb.

- If you use a stand magnifier (one that sits directly on the page), you'll need a clipboard, a lap desk, or ideally a variable-height pull-up table on casters that can hold a reading stand. You can use the same table along with good lighting for writing or projects. Alternatively, you may find it easier to read at a table you already own. If so, consider purchasing a comfortable desk chair to match.

- If you use a CCTV, you may need a pair of glasses just for reading with your machine to see optimally. Your bifocals may not work because you need to look straight at the machine and the bifocals are designed for you to look down while you're reading. If you're nearsighted, try taking your glasses off when you use your CCTV.

TIPS FOR AUDIO READING

- Mark the little black buttons on your electronics, including the on-off and play buttons on your tape player, with contrasting-colored tape or puff paint.

- If you have hearing loss, consider choosing taped books, magazines, and papers narrated by men, since their voices are usually easier to hear than women's higher-pitched voices.

- For enhancing your hearing or listening quietly while others are in the room, try a personal amplifier headset or regular headset.

- Consider purchasing a four-track tape player in order to listen to NLS and other free recordings on a smaller, more portable player than the one provided with your NLS membership (the LS&S catalog has the best selection).

Knitting, Sewing, and Projects

- To have good light and magnification and still have both hands free, use a gooseneck floor lamp with a mounted magnifier that can be placed next to your work and adjusted as necessary. Be sure to check the power of these magnifiers against your own magnification needs when ordering. You can also use them in combination with reading glasses.

- For knitting, use color-contrasting needles and yarn. Knit or crochet with dark needles and light yarn or light needles and darker yarn. Place a solid-color contrasting cloth or towel underneath your work for better visibility. Avoid working with pastels or colors you have difficulty seeing.

- Use a self-threading needle stuck into a bar of soap for stability and thread your needle by touch. Sew dark buttons with white thread and use a dark permanent marker afterward to color the thread. Sew on a contrasting-color tablecloth in order to see the thread.

Mail

If your mailbox is located a significant distance from your front door and it's difficult or unsafe to walk there and back (which can happen in winter when the walks are icy), ask your doctor for a letter stating that you cannot drive and are unable to pick up your mail. Your postal carrier will deliver your mail to your door.

PRODUCT SUGGESTIONS

Large-print and audio books, newspapers, and magazines

Giant-button television and VCR remote

Talking VCR player

Television screen enlarger

Self-threading needles

Color-contrasting knitting needles and yarn

Hands-free magnifiers

Big-print or talking measuring tape

Large-print checks, address book, and date book

Medium-thick black felt-tip pen

White unlined or darkly lined paper

Voice-activated PDA or electronic organizer

Talking or jumbo-display calculator

Large-button large-print phone with voice-activated dialing

Talking or jumbo-faced watch

Talking or large-print clock

CCTV

Screen enlargement and talking computer software

Bills, Letters, and Home Offices

Between computer software, talking office machines, CCTVs, large-print checks, and a host of other products, you can create a home office that enables you to do virtually any daily business you'd like. Here a few suggestions:

TIPS FOR BILLS, CHECKS, AND BANKING

- You can order large-print checks and check registers from your bank. Large-print checks fit easily into standard-sized legal envelopes.

- The easiest way to approach reading bills is to scan in the most predictable places for the key information: the company, the amount, and the due date. You can use any variety of magnifiers or a CCTV to do this (see chapter 12). The company name is almost always at the top of the first page, either on the right or left or in the center. The amount is usually on the right-hand side of the first page, often in bold type. The date may be anywhere, but it will be in the same place for each company every month. Some companies provide large-print statements as a courtesy if you request them. You can also opt for automatic payment from your bank account, especially for utility bills.

- If you prefer regular-sized checks, choose a plain design with black type on a white background. Avoid checks with flowers, pictures, or pastel colors. You can use a check-writing guide to make sure your writing stays on the right lines.

- For writing checks, try using a lamp magnifier like the Big Eye and high-power reading glasses at half the strength you normally need to read. Lower-strength glasses will give you a more comfortable writing distance and should still work well for writing, since you do not need to see quite as clearly to write as you do to read.

- Use a talking calculator to reconcile your statement or checkbook or combine personal banking software with screen enlargement or talking computer software for on-line banking.

TIPS FOR PHONE CALLS

- Use a large-print address book and make entries in block letters large enough to read easily with a medium-thick black felt-tip pen. Alternatively, make your own address or phone list in large print from your computer. You can make your electronic address book portable with a voice-activated

Parrot PDA or Voice Diary electronic organizer, featured in the low-vision product catalogs in appendix C.

- When you take messages or handwrite notes for yourself, always use a medium-thick black felt-tip pen, never ballpoint pens, colored pens, or pencils, which are too difficult to see. Always write on white paper, not colored or cream paper.

- Choose a big-button telephone with good color contrast from the many offered in the low-vision product catalogs listed in appendix C. Do not buy a white phone with gray numbers, which are too hard to see.

- You may also want a phone with automatic voice-activated dialing or an amplifier feature for easier listening. Alternatively, program your speed-dial function for routine numbers and create a large-print directory or map of your speed-dial pad or mark your automatic dialing buttons with color-coded tape, permanent markers, or puff paint.

- There are a number of other low-vision phone products on the market, including a remote-controlled speakerphone with voice-activated answering, a Backtalk dialing accessory that tells you which number you've just dialed, and a talking caller ID machine.

- Use your phone company's automated message service. It's often easier to operate and sounds clearer than a home answering machine.

TIPS FOR TIME AND APPOINTMENTS

- Avoid digital clocks and watches with poorly visible displays. Choose a talking or jumbo-faced watch from the dozens of styles available, and opt for large-print black-and-white room clocks or talking clocks. Put one in each room as needed.

- Use a large-print date book and a medium-thick black felt-tip pen for appointment entries or use a voice-activated Parrot PDA or Voice Diary electronic organizer.

TIPS FOR COMPUTERS

- Consult with your local visual rehabilitation center, the members of MD Support, and the computer retailers listed in appendix C to determine the best combination of hardware and software for you. You may also want to consider upgrading to a large, high-resolution monitor with good backlighting. See chapter 12 for a longer discussion.

YOU DON'T NEED TO BE HELEN KELLER

Not everyone with low vision wants to try skydiving, set up a home office, fly across the country, cook a four-course meal for family and friends, or even write his or her own checks. Just because all of these things can be done with low vision doesn't mean you have to do them. Visual rehabilitation is about having the life that will make you the happiest and determining for yourself what that might be.

FOR YOUR KITCHEN AND DINING ROOM

Kitchens can easily become cluttered. Before you start cooking, clear away as much as you can, discard unused jars, and avoid overstuffing your shelves. Organize your kitchen so that everything has its place and is easy for you to find. It's more important to see what you have than to have a lot that you can't see. Make sure you have clearly lit counter space. Ceiling lights are almost never good enough. Try installing fluorescent lighting underneath your counter (as long as it doesn't glare into your eyes) or use a countertop gooseneck adjustable lamp with an indoor floodlight bulb. Use dish towels or place mats to cut countertop glare.

GENERAL COOKING TIPS

- Buy a selection of large-print cookbooks or make your own by reprinting your favorite recipes in a medium-width black felt-tip marker on 8.5-by-11-inch paper and collecting them in a handy binder. Enlarge the recipes in chapter 4 on a photocopy machine and add them to your collection.

- Use color contrast whenever you can. Prepare onions, potatoes, cauliflower, garlic, mushrooms, chicken, and whitefish on a dark cutting board. Prepare dark leafy greens, red and green peppers, celery, carrots, beef, pork, and salmon on a white cutting board.

- Mark your microwave and stove dials with puff paint, contrasting-color tape, or Braille.

- Consider using a talking kitchen scale, talking cooking thermometer, safety spatula, or any of the many other products offered in low-vision catalogs for the kitchen.

- Consider grouping items you are cooking on a plastic tray with sides to keep them handy and organized, especially if you are working with small amounts of hard-to-see foods.

- Use your sense of smell and touch and your experience to guide you.

TIPS FOR POURING AND MEASURING

- To minimize spills, set your cup, glass, pitcher, or bowl in the sink when you pour. When pouring from a container, rest the lip of the container on the edge of the glass for more stability. Don't fill glasses or cups to the top. Use coffee mugs with lids.

- With cold liquids, slip your finger over the edge of the glass and stop pouring when the liquid reaches your finger. With hot liquids, consider using a beeping liquid level indicator.

- Drink coffee from a white mug and milk from a dark glass.

- Use a big-print measuring cup or mark your measuring cup with black permanent marker. Use a multicolored measuring spoon or cup set to distinguish between different amounts, or mark your measuring equipment with different-colored stickers or large-print numbers.

TIPS FOR STOVES AND OVENS

- Mark the dials or buttons of your appliances, especially the ones you use the most frequently, with a black permanent marker, contrasting-color tape, puff paint, or Braille.

- Check new appliances for visibility before purchasing them. Sometimes fancy digital appliances are much harder to see than cheaper models.

- Use oven mitts instead of handheld hotpads to reduce the risk of accidental burns. Always pull the oven rack out before you remove pans. Listen for a click or double-check your appliances when you turn them off.

TIPS FOR DINING

- Buy solid-color formal china and smash your flowered ones. (Just kidding. See Zelda Grant's story in chapter 5.) Buy two inexpensive place settings for daily use: one in a light color and the other in a dark color. Use them interchangeably for contrast with different foods. For example, eat mashed potatoes and whitefish on a dark plate and steak and dark green salad on a light plate.

- Eat foods that run away easily, such as peas and corn, from bowls, as you would with fruits such as blueberries.

- Buy solid-color tablecloths with good color contrast against your dishes.

FOR YOUR BEDROOM AND BATH

As in the kitchen, using contrast to your advantage can be really helpful in the bedroom and bath. Good lighting is, of course, important, too, especially in closets and bathrooms, where glare can be a problem.

TIPS FOR CLOTHING

- Carry your clothing choices into the sunlight during the day, where color differences will be more visible, and make your decision then.

- Upgrade the lighting in your closet or use a handheld flashlight or lighted hand magnifier.

- Feel for clothing tags to tell if items are right side out and facing forward.

- Keep similarly colored clothes separated in your closet and labeled with safety pins. For example, put one pin in navy clothes, two in green clothes, and none in black clothes. Use brightly colored storage drawers to separate similarly colored socks or sweaters.

- Consider choosing one base color, such as navy blue, brown, or black, and designing your seasonal wardrobes around this color for ease and flexibility.

- Use a flashlight or clip-on gooseneck lamp to see washing machine and dryer dials. Label them with permanent markers, colored tape, puff paint, or Braille.

- Tell your dry cleaner you have low vision and ask him or her to group your clothing by color and tell you if there are any spots left. If so, discard that item. If your cleaner is unresponsive, try arriving at a slow time of day or choose another cleaner who is friendlier.

- Wear an oven mitt when ironing and never iron with poor lighting. Use a contrasting ironing board cover or a towel to make clothing more visible. Iron in a regular pattern (from left to right or top to bottom).

TIPS FOR PUTTIN' ON THE DOG

- Use a magnifying makeup mirror. Consider arranging with your husband, neighbor, or friend to tell you whether you've gotten your makeup the way you like it.

- Try an electric shaver and use your fingers to feel for areas you've missed. When you find an area, place your opposite finger next to it and bring the shaver up to meet it.

- Rest your hand on a contrasting-color cloth and use a gooseneck lamp with an attached magnifier for clipping nails. Use Easy Hold clippers rather than scissors.

- Organize your bath and vanity table so that everything has its place and everything is either easy to see or clearly labeled. You may want to use brightly colored organizer trays to keep items separate.

- Design your bath with color contrast in mind. If it's white, use solid dark primary-colored towels, toothbrushes, a darker toothpaste tube, and a dark soap tray. Use the bathroom mirror for styling your hair and hang a solid-colored towel behind your head for contrast. If you have dark hair, hang a light towel; if you have light hair, hang a dark towel.

TIPS FOR STAYING SAFE AND HEALTHY

- Avoid using toxic substances such as powerful bleaches and pesticides. We don't usually need those chemicals to have a clean home and healthy plants.

- Plug in cords by placing one finger against the outlet and aiming the plug with the other hand. If it doesn't fit, feel for the position of the prongs and try again. If this doesn't work, bring in a gooseneck lamp with a floodlight bulb or a high-powered flashlight and try to get your eyes down to the level of the plug.

- Mark your preferred temperatures on your thermostat or purchase a boldface thermostat dial or a big-print or talking thermostat.

- Mark medicine bottles with puff paint, colored tape, rubber bands, or easily visible permanent marker. Keep medicines that are easily confused in different rooms or on different shelves.

- Keep a set of large white index cards, one for each prescription you have. Using a black felt-tip marker, write down the prescription information for one medication on each card with as many slash marks as there are refills. As you reorder, cross each slash mark so that you always know how many refills you have left. Keep your index cards together in a box or on a ring.

PRODUCT SUGGESTIONS

Large-print cookbooks

Contrasting solid-color dishes and tablecloths

Large-print, talking, or beeping kitchen utensils and appliances

Magnifying mirror

Color-contrasting towels, toothbrush, and soap tray

Talking weight scale, blood pressure meter, and thermometer

Big-print pillboxes

Big-print insulin syringes and syringe magnifiers

Large-print thermostat dial or talking thermostat

SAVING SIGHT IN YOUR COMMUNITY

Life is a daring adventure! It gives us back only as much as we risk. Leave your self-consciousness in your closet and take your courage and confidence with you. Venturing out of the house always entails risk. But no one in the world cares about whether we make mistakes except us. If we can make them freely, with patience and humor, we allow others to relax, too. The tips in this section are designed to be read along with chapter 13, which talks about driving, walking, and transportation, and chapter 6, which discusses social interactions, taking risks, and building connections to your community.

The Magic of White Canes

White identification canes are like magic. They increase your safety on the street by alerting motorists that you may not see them. White canes also have a salutary effect on people. They encourage altruistic behavior, and they discourage impatience. A white cane can be a tremendously effective way to say "I have low vision" without having to explain, and people almost always respond positively. We are often reluctant to use white canes, fearing vulnerability. But the American Foundation for the Blind reports that carrying a white cane does not increase your risk of crime.

You may be thinking, *What? Me with a white cane? You've got to be kidding!* Many of my patients tell me exactly that. We so closely associate white canes with being completely blind or appearing conspicuous that carrying one does not usually fit our self-image. But it works. It really does. And many of the very same patients who were ready to fire me as their doctor when I suggested a white cane now swear by it, even if they only use it at dusk, for crossing major intersections, or in airports.

White identification canes are only for signaling others, particularly drivers, not for tapping sidewalks or supporting your weight. They are shorter than the canes used by the blind and lighter than regular canes used for walking support. They come in lightweight foldable models that you can carry in a purse, bag, or briefcase and use when needed.

Low-Vision Buttons

A low-profile alternative to a white cane is an I HAVE LOW VISION button. Keep one with you and pin it to your coat or sweater when you travel, shop, or dine out. We give them away at our program in Michigan and they've been very popular. You can order a button from the National Association for the Visually Handicapped (NAVH) at 212-889-3141 or from Ann Morris Enterprises at 800-454-3175.

Leaving Home

• Our front walks, porches, and foyers are often dark, which makes keyholes hard to see and alarms hard to operate, and it isn't safe. You may want to install outdoor floodlights on the porch and indoor floodlights in the foyer. Consider putting your outdoor lights on timers or motion sensors so that they are always on when you need them the most.

- Carry a pocket magnifier and a high-powered penlight or small flashlight with you for reading menus, bills, and price tags. Backcountry camping stores may be better sources for these lights than hardware stores, which tend to sell bulkier models.

- Keys often look alike. Label your look-alike keys with brightly colored key covers or safety pins. Put the key you use most often on the outside of the ring.

- To help aim your key, put one finger on the keyhole and aim toward that finger.

- If the buttons on your home alarm are hard to see, label them with puff paint. Sometimes it's difficult to remember alarm combinations or keypad configurations. Try making a large-print map of the keypad with a black felt-tip marker on a white sheet of paper. Hang this paper on the wall next to the alarm.

Money

- Arrange your bills in a multicompartment billfold and insert the bills upside down so the big-print numbers are visible. Or you can fold them in identifying patterns. For example, keep one-dollar bills straight, fold five-dollar bills in half horizontally so they are long and thin, fold ten-dollar bills in half vertically so they are square, and fold twenty-dollar bills at the right corner. Avoid carrying larger bills whenever possible.

- Memorize the sizes and shapes of coins. Quarters and dimes have ridged edges, but quarters are much larger. Nickels and pennies have smooth edges, but nickels are much thicker and heavier. The new one-dollar coins are as large as quarters, but they have smooth edges.

- If you have several pockets, keep pennies in one, quarters in another, and nickels and dimes in a third. Alternatively, use a multicompartment change purse.

Shopping

- If your schedule is flexible, shop at off-peak hours so that you don't have the hassle of crowds and the clerks are less stressed and have time to be more helpful.

- If you're looking for a particular item, consider calling the store ahead of time to see if it's in stock. Ask them to hold it for you at the counter.

- Take your pocket flashlight, penlight, or lighted magnifier to see price tags.

- Make it a habit to double-check your purchases with the clerk to ensure that you've got the right size, color, and product. Ask about restricted return policies, which are often printed on small unreadable signs at the register.

- Memorize the layout of your favorite grocery store and the labels of your favorite brands.

- Consider asking your grocer whether they offer a delivery service, take telephone orders for pickup, or can assist you while you shop in the store if you call ahead and arrange a time.

- Make a large-print grocery list with a black felt-tip pen on white paper. Arrange the items according to the layout of the store. Alternatively, create a large-print grocery check-off list on your computer that you can use every week.

Dining Out

- If your schedule is flexible, dine at off-peak hours when you're more likely to get better service and less pressure to rush through your meal.

- Choose well-lit restaurants and request a table with the best lighting for you (which may actually be a darker area if you are extremely glare-sensitive). Sit with your back to the window or light source to maximize the light on your menu and plate and minimize glare.

- Use your penlight or lighted handheld magnifier to read menus. You can also request a large-print menu from the waitstaff or request that they read you the selections. Federal law mandates that restaurants be accessible to people with low vision, so you are entitled to equal access to the menu.

- Consider borrowing menus from your favorite restaurants, and browsing them ahead of time with a magnifier or on your CCTV or enlarging them on a copy machine for easier reading. You can do the same with carry-out menus.

- When your food arrives, do not hesitate to ask your waiter to tell you exactly what is on your plate and where it is. You may want to say that you have low vision so that he or she understands your request and can be helpful identifying other things that are hard to see, such as the right restroom door and the numbers on the bill.

Parties

Remember that people come to parties to meet you and enjoy your company. They are usually much more concerned about feeling comfortable themselves and appearing attractive than about whether or not you have low vision. And you have much more to offer at a party than how much you can or can't see. Introduce yourself freely and tell people that you will not be able to recognize their faces so they must introduce themselves in return.

- Put yourself and your host at ease by communicating directly. Feel free to ask for a bowl or a plate with a rim for hors d'oeuvres if you'd be more comfortable with one. Do not hesitate to ask for guided directions to the bar or bathroom.

- Ask your friends to play with large-print cards, which are the same size as regular cards and are easier for everyone to see.

- For regular card games, bring a portable gooseneck lamp with a floodlight bulb for the playing table.

Remember that friends want your company, not perfect vision, and clubs are for members, including you. Living with low vision means letting the world know what you need and helping people meet those needs. When you feel comfortable, everyone around you will feel more comfortable, too.

PRODUCT SUGGESTIONS

White identification cane

Multicompartment billfold and change purse

Large-print playing cards and Uno, Rook, and bingo cards

Large-print Scrabble and Monopoly

Uniquely shaped high-contrast poker chips

Uniquely shaped high-contrast chess and checker sets

Binoculars and monocular lenses

Sports and Exercise

While there are some sports or forms of exercise, such as tennis, that don't work very well with low vision, there are others, such as golf, bowling, walking, swimming, pool running, yoga, tai chi, and Exercycling, that do. Always be sure to check with your doctor before you change your physical routine, and don't assume that low vision means you can't be active (see chapter 6).

- For golf, use your experience and body alignment to guide your stroke. Use your binoculars or monocular to see the putting green, or ask a friend to stand by the hole for better visibility. On courses that still allow caddies, retain one to identify your ball or ask your friends.

- For bowling, aim for the black lane markers and consider using a slightly lighter ball for easier handling. Use your binoculars or monocular telescope to read the screen or see the pins, or ask a teammate.

- Don't opt out just because you decide to forgo the sports part of an event. Meet your friends for lunch after their tennis match. Go fishing or hunting with your buddies regardless. Sports aren't only about hitting little balls or pins, casting little hooks, or firing guns. They're about sharing an experience,

relaxing together, and shooting the breeze.
You can do that with the best of them.

Music and Religious Services

- If you play an instrument, enlarge your sheet
  music on a copy machine, order big-print
  copies, or borrow large-print music through
  the NLS Music Service (see appendix B).

- Increase the amount of light shining directly
  on your score by using a gooseneck clip or
  stand lamp with an indoor floodlight, or
  position your music stand at home for
  optimal sunlight.

- Try a Walter's hands-free magnifier
  headband with the low-powered lens option
  for piano playing (make sure it's returnable
  if it doesn't work for you).

- Call your place of worship and ask which
  hymns they plan to sing. Enlarge those
  pages from your hymnal on a copy machine
  and take them with you to services. You can
  also enlarge the entire program or ask your
  clergy to E-mail it to you ahead of time so
  you can print it out in large font.
  Alternatively, ask your church to publish
  their program in large print on a regular
  basis. There are probably a number of other
  people in the congregation who can't read a

standard font, either, especially if it's written in script or printed on colored paper.

- If you sing in the choir, arrange for large-print copies of the music from your choirmaster. You can also use a small high-powered handheld penlight or a clip light on your music book or stand for better visibility.

- Tell your friends, clergy, and other congregation members that you cannot recognize faces and that you would love to greet them, but they need to identify themselves. Consider volunteering as a greeter for some services so that everyone gets to know you and you have a chance to say hello.

- If it's too far to walk to services and the bus doesn't go there, tell your clergy that you need a ride. Many churches have free rides available. Or organize shared rides with other members who have low vision or would rather not drive alone. Alternatively, ask another member who lives near you for a regular ride and take him or her out every once in a while for lunch or dinner.

Working and Volunteering

Do not assume that vision loss means unemployment or an inability to volunteer effectively or be active in your community. Seniors with low vision work as attorneys, professors, company owners, political activists, counselors, hospital and church greeters, patient visitors, reading tutors, and much more. See chapter 6 for volunteering ideas and advice for approaching your colleagues, friends, and neighborhood organizations with confidence. See appendix D for more information on the Americans with Disabilities Act (ADA) and your rights to equal treatment in the workplace and in public establishments.

WELCOME HOME

Welcome home and congratulations on finishing this rehabilitation program! Tuck your keys in their regular place and give yourself some credit for having gone out and done whatever you needed or wanted to do in the world. Sometimes visual rehabilitation can feel overwhelming, especially if you've only recently lost vision or if you are experiencing depression. But keep going! Reach out to the resources that you have in this book, in the appendixes, in your community, with your family and friends, and within yourself. Keep your heart and your humor. We're rooting for you. You can do it.

PART IV:

Appendixes and Index

Macular Degeneration Organizations, Finding Visual Rehabilitation Programs in Your Area, On-line Communities, and Memoirs by People with Vision Loss

MACULAR DEGENERATION ORGANIZATIONS

The Association for Macular Diseases
Under the leadership of Nikolai Stevenson, who
has age-related macular degeneration, the
association offers a large-print quarterly
newsletter with research updates and articles and
other services, including free seminars throughout
the United States. Thousands of members
worldwide. For membership information contact:
212-605-3719
association@retinalresearch.org
www.macula.org

Macular Degeneration International

Founded by Tom Perski, who has Stargardt's disease (the juvenile form of macular degeneration), MDI offers a large-print biannual news journal with research updates, information on participating in clinical trials, and a toll-free help line. Holds free seminars throughout the United States. Thousands of members worldwide. For membership information contact:
800-393-7634
info@maculardegeneration.org
www.maculardegeneration.org

Macular Degeneration Partnership

Los Angeles–based coalition of patients, professionals in low vision, and physicians who work to educate doctors and the public about macular degeneration and low-vision rehabilitation. Provides a monthly on-line newsletter and an E-mail subscription service, AMD Update. Will answer additional questions by E-mail through the Web site, or call toll-free to leave a message and hear recorded information.
888-430-9898
www.amd.org

FINDING ALL OF YOUR VISUAL REHABILITATION OPTIONS

There are six ways to find visual rehabilitation programs in your area (Canadians see appendix F):

1. Ask your doctor for a referral (although he or she may not know about local programs).

2. Visit Directory of Services at the American Foundation for the Blind (AFB) Web site.

3. Contact the VA if you are a veteran.

4. Call your state Commission for the Blind.

5. Contact the macular degeneration organizations listed earlier.

6. Post a query about visual rehabilitation through MD Support (see "On-line Communities").
   Note: You may be eligible for several programs, some of which are free of charge. *None of these sources will know about all of the programs available to you, so you need to contact each of them to really know all of your options for visual rehabilitation.*

FINDING VISUAL REHABILITATION PROGRAMS IN YOUR AREA

American Foundation for the Blind (AFB)
Provides an excellent on-line *Directory of Services* that lists all of the visual rehabilitation programs nationwide. You can search by state for listings in your area. The directory does not distinguish between programs that vary greatly in scope and quality (See chapter 9 for a guide to choosing visual rehabilitation programs), so you should check out all of the programs in your area. You can also call the AFB directly and ask for the listings.
800-232-5463 (nationwide)
312-245-9961 (Chicago office)
415-392-4845 (San Francisco office)
214-352-7222 (Dallas office)
404-525-2303 (Atlanta office)
afbinfo@afb.net
www.afb.org

United States Department of Veterans Affairs
VA programs often provide excellent training, although sometimes they are geared to younger adults. Call the health care benefits phone line below. They will refer you to the nearest VA facility for eligibility assessment and referral.
General VA Benefits: 800-827-1000
VA Low-Vision Benefits: 877-222-8387
www.va.gov/blindrehab

Your State Commission for the Blind

State commissions often have excellent free or low-cost visual rehabilitation programs, although they may be geared primarily toward younger adults. South Dakota and Utah have particularly good services. Visit your state government's home page or call your local state representative or senator and ask for the phone number for your state commission.

ON-LINE COMMUNITIES

Brian's Eye Story
by Brian Harron
www.brianseye.com

Judy's Jolts of Hope
by Judy Prevost
www.total.net/~judyp/

Linda's Macular Degeneration Hope Page
by Linda Olsen
www.geocities.com/linda1958.geo

MD Support
A vibrant on-line community founded by Dan Roberts, who has low vision from a macular condition. Join MDList, an E-mail group with more than 450 members around the world, or post a question to the MD Support Internet

message board. MD Support also offers a Web library of articles, links, research updates, and two new informational videos, *Macular Degeneration: The Inside Story* and *The T.A.S.K. of Living with Central Vision Loss.*
director@mdsupport.org
www.mdsupport.org

MEMOIRS BY PEOPLE WITH VISION LOSS

Free audiotaped copies of these memoirs may be available through the National Library Service (NLS) or Canadian National Institute for the Blind (CNIB) Library Books on Tape programs (see appendix B and appendix F, respectively). Ask your bookstore about regular and large-print editions.

By Younger Adults
Hull, John. *Touching the Rock.* New York: Pantheon, 1990.

Kleege, Georgina. *Sight Unseen.* New Haven: Yale University Press, 1999.

Kuusisto, Stephen. *Planet of the Blind.* New York: Dial, 1998.

Pey, Tom. *Bang! You're Dead.* New York: John Wiley & Sons, 2001.

By Older Adults

Grunwald, Henry. *Twilight: Losing Sight, Gaining Insight.* New York: Knopf, 1999.

Neer, Frances Lief. *Dancing in the Dark.* Berkeley, CA: Creative Arts, 1994.

———, editor. *Perceiving the Elephant.* Berkeley, CA: Creative Arts, 1998.

See, Carolyn. "Going Blind and Fighting in Every Possible Way." *Modern Maturity,* September–October 1997, 47–49.

Silverman, Bert. *Bert's Eye View: Coping with Macular Degeneration* (guidebook with autobiographical vignettes). Portland, ME: Viewpoint Press, 1997.

Wason, Betty. *Macular Degeneration: Living Positively with Vision Loss* (guidebook with biographical vignettes). Alameda, CA: Hunter House, 1998.

Reading, Watching, and Listening

WATCHING TV AND VIDEO

Descriptive Video Service (DVS)
WGBH Boston, MA
A free nationwide service that provides a clear descriptive narration to accompany movies and PBS shows on television so that you can easily follow and enjoy the programs. All you need is a stereo TV with a Second Audio Program feature (SAP), a VCR with SAP, or an SAP receiver that can be used with or without a TV. Most TVs and VCRs built since 1998 come with this feature. To hear the narration, simply consult your user's manual to activate the SAP feature. Contact WGBH for a schedule of narrated programs or to purchase videos with DVS for about fifteen dollars each. DVS videos are also available at many public libraries.
800-333-1203 (automated information)
617-300-3490

BROADCAST NEWSSTANDS

In Touch Networks
A subsidiary of the Jewish Guild for the Blind, In Touch broadcasts eight hours of articles read from major magazines and newspapers daily; broadcast recycles three times for twenty-four-hour listening. Service nationwide in the United States to people of any faith who have visual or physical impairments that impede reading. Doctor's letter required. Onetime membership fee of $125 covers radio with special receiving microchip and lifetime service. Free membership for Medicaid recipients.
212-769-6270 (New York City)
800-456-3166 (nationwide)
intouchinfo@jgb.org
www.intouchnetworks.org

National Public Radio
Your local public radio station offers a wide range of very high-quality national and international news and feature programs that closely parallel the coverage in the *New York Times* and other papers. Also features many shows on science, money, music, current events, entertainment, and more. Tune in on your radio dial between FM 87 and FM 92 or visit their Web site and click on "find a station" for one in your area.
www.npr.org

Radio Reading Service

Free broadcast reading of local and major newspapers and national magazines. Programming varies by community; not available everywhere. Call your local public radio station or university radio station for information about your area.

LEARNING BRAILLE

The Hadley School for the Blind

A well-respected correspondence school based in Winnetka, Illinois, that offers free self-paced Braille classes for people with vision loss and their family and friends worldwide. Hadley is currently developing a special course for seniors using jumbo-sized Braille. Call or E-mail to request a large-print catalog or download one from their Web site.
800-323-4238
info@hadley-school.org
www.hadley-school.org

LARGE-PRINT BOOKS, PERIODICALS, AND MUSIC

Large print is usually a sixteen-point font. You will probably be able to read large print if you have good contrast sensitivity and 20/100 vision or better. If large print is too hard to see, see the wonderful selection of free books, magazines, and newspapers on audiotape listed in "Free Audio-taped Books and Periodicals."

Amazon.com
Choose from more than 7,000 titles in large print, all genres. Type in keywords "large print books" in Amazon.com's site search window. Prices vary.
www.amazon.com

Doubleday Large Print Book Club
Mail-order book club for large-print books. Choose from a wide selection of best-sellers by authors such as John Grisham and Danielle Steele, mysteries, romances, and literature.
800-688-4442
www.doubledaylargeprint.com

The National Association for the Visually Handicapped (NAVH)
Free by-mail lending library of 7,000 titles in large print; ships books nationwide in the United States only. Also offers quarterly newsletter with membership. Retail store for low-vision products at 22 West 21st Street, 6th Floor, in Manhattan.
212-889-3141
staff@navh.org
www.navh.org

National Library Service (NLS) Music Service

Free national lending library for large-print and Braille scores for voice, piano, and other instruments. Also provides music magazines, opera librettos, biographies of popular and classical musicians, and general music histories. Service to all fifty states and Americans living in Canada.
800-424-8567
202-707-0712 (Washington, D.C.)
nlsm@loc.gov
www.loc.gov/nls

The New York Times Large Type Weekly

The best articles from each week's *Times*, including national news, health, business, the arts, sports, and the crossword puzzle.
800-631-2580
www.nytimes.com/nytstore/publications

Reader's Digest Large Edition

Reader's Digest's large-print edition comes on easy-to-read nonglare paper. A one-year subscription costs roughly twenty dollars. *Reader's Digest* can also transfer your current regular subscription to the large edition.
800-807-2780
www.rd.com/store

Thorndike Press

Offers a large selection of large-print books, all genres. Prices vary. Call for a large-print catalog.
800-877-4253
www.gale.com/thorndike

FREE AUDIOTAPED BOOKS AND PERIODICALS

American Printing House for the Blind (APH)

Free audiotaped subscription to *Reader's Digest* and *Newsweek* for American citizens living in the fifty states or Canada. Canadians may purchase subscriptions for roughly the cost of a regular-print subscription. Requires a four-track tape player (your NLS or CNIB player will work). Also offers large-print, computer file, and Braille publications.
800-223-1839
info@aph.org
www.aph.org

Choice Magazine Listening

Offers free bimonthly four-track cassette tapes with eight hours of unabridged magazine articles, fiction, and poetry read by professional actors. The tapes are yours to keep; no return necessary. Play them on a free NLS player or purchase your own four-track tape player from a low-vision catalog.

Subscriptions and shipping within the fifty states only or to American citizens living in Canada.
516-883-8280 (New York)
888-724-6423 (888-7-CHOICE)
choicemag@aol.com
www.choicemagazinelistening.org

Jewish Guild for the Blind (JGB)
Free by-mail autotape lending library featuring more than 1,600 unabridged works of popular fiction, romance, and nonfiction. New titles announced regularly. Return postage free as material for the blind. Ships worldwide to people of any faith with vision loss.
212-769-6331
audiolibrary@jgb.org
www.jgb.org

National Library Service (NLS) Library of Congress Talking Book Program
The Library of Congress has a fantastic lending program of thousands of books on tape by mail. Return postage is free. The tapes can only be played on a four-track tape player, which the library also provides on indefinite loan. Amplified headphones available for the hard-of-hearing. Go to the NLS Web site or call their 800 number for more information. Applications available at your county library. Doctor's signature required. Available nationwide and to American citizens living in Canada.

202-707-5100 (Washington, D.C.)

800-424-8567 (nationwide in the U.S.)

www.loc.gov/nls

National Library Service (NLS) Magazine Program

Borrow your favorite magazine on tape. Includes the *Atlantic Monthly, Discover, Good Housekeeping, National Geographic,* the *New York Times Book Review, Reader's Digest* (also in Spanish), *Sports Illustrated, US News and World Report,* and many others. See above for application information.

800-424-8567

www.loc.gov/nls

PURCHASING AN NLS- OR CNIB-COMPATIBLE FOUR-TRACK TAPE PLAYER

This is not necessary, since you can borrow one from the NLS (American) or CNIB (Canadian) for free. But these machines are bulky and meant only for use at home. If you travel, would like to carry one around town, or own a player, you can choose from a variety of smaller models from the LS&S catalog or another low-vision catalog (see appendix C).

Recording for the Blind and Dyslexic (RFBD)

Free or low-cost audiotaped textbooks and educational materials for any class you would like to take. Makes going back to school possible. Ships worldwide.
800-221-4792
www.rfbd.org

AUDIOTAPED AND LARGE-PRINT RELIGIOUS WORKS

American Bible Society (retail bookstore)

Offers the King James Version, Good News, and Reina Valera Spanish Bibles in large print and audiotape through their on-line store. Prices vary. Retail bookstore at 1865 Broadway in Manhattan.
800-322-4253
www.americanbible.org
www.bibles.com (on-line store)

Aurora Ministries (nondenominational)

Through its Audio Scripture Ministry, Aurora Ministries gives a free Bible on cassette tape in any of sixty-four different languages to anyone with vision loss or physical impairments that impede reading. Choose between the New King James Version (NKJV) and traditional King James Version (KJV). Ships worldwide. No return necessary.

941-748-3031
tapes@auroraministries.org
www.gospelcom.net/aurora

Christian Book (retail bookstore)

Offers fiction, music, videos, Christian living
publications, and thousands of Bibles, including
large-print, giant-print, and supergiant-print
versions. Prices vary.
508-977-5000
orders@christianbook.com
www.christianbook.com

Christian Record Services (nondenominational)

Provides free Christian magazine subscriptions
in large print and audiotape. Free by-mail
lending library features 1,700 audiotaped and
Braille books; return postage free as material for
the blind. Also sells gift and study Bibles; prices
vary. Subscriptions and shipping worldwide.
402-488-0981
info@christianrecord.org
www.christianrecord.org

Dar-us-Salam Publications (retail publisher)

Offers the Qur'an on audiotape and CD-ROM in
Arabic. Some versions have English translations.
Also offers a wide variety of other popular and
religious works in various languages and

formats. Prices vary. Retail bookstore at 1111
Conrad Sauer Drive in Houston.
713-722-0419
sales@dar-us-salam.com
www.dar-us-salam.com

The Jewish Braille Institute of America (unaffiliated)

Free by-mail lending library of more than 10,000
audiotaped, large-print, and Braille popular
works with Jewish themes or authors and
religious books in Hebrew and English. Also
offers gift-quality large-print religious works.
Ships worldwide to people of any faith with visual
or physical impairments that impede reading.
212-889-2525 (New York City)
800-433-1531 (nationwide)
admin@jbilibrary.org
www.jbilibrary.org

Lutheran Library for the Blind (Missouri Synod)

Free by-mail lending library featuring 4,000
large-print, audiotaped, and Braille books and
publications, including the Lutheran catechism,
hymnals, and Lutheran magazines. Service to
continental United States and Canada; return
postage free as material for the blind.
800-433-3954
blind.mission@lcms.org
www.blindmission.org

Xavier Society for the Blind (Roman Catholic)

Free by-mail lending library of Roman Catholic spiritual and inspirational books and magazines, including the *Catholic Review*. Over 1,000 publications to choose from. Ships throughout North America. Return postage free as material for the blind.

212-473-7800 (New York City)

800-637-9193 (nationwide)

The Best Low-Vision Product Catalogs, and CCTVs, Computers, and Software

THE BEST LOW-VISION PRODUCT CATALOGS

Independent Living Aids (ILA)
Beautiful color pictures, clear explanations in bold print, and a very good selection. Call for a free catalog:
800-537-2118
can-do@independentliving.com
www.independentliving.com

LS&S Group
Excellent selection with good customer service. Catalog recently redesigned with bold print for easier reading. Co-owned by John Bace, who has macular degeneration. Includes Bace's "Father's Favorite" column of recommended products. Call for a free catalog:
800-468-4789
info@lssonline.net
www.lssgroup.com

Maxi Aids
Warehouse-style catalog with tiny pictures and dense print but a very wide selection. Call for a free catalog:
800-522-6294
sales@maxiaids.com
www.maxiaids.com

The National Association of the Visually Handicapped (NAVH)
Smaller selection with good descriptions in large print. Call for a free catalog:
415-221-3201 (Western and Mountain states)
212-889-3141 (all other states and Canada)
staff@navh.org
www.navh.org

NOIR (sunglasses)
Choose amber-colored lenses or call NOIR for information on which lenses will best block blue light and reduce glare. Lenses clip onto or fit over your regular glasses.
800-521-9746
www.noir-medical.com

BATTERY-POWERED SCOOTERS

Amigo Mobility International
800-692-6446 (800-MY-AMIGO)
info@myamigo.com
www.myamigo.com

Electric Mobility
800-662-4548 (800-MOBILITY)
800-665-0065 (Canada)
800-878-3855 (U.S. Veterans)
in_home@electricmobility.com
veterans@electricmobility.com (U.S. Veterans)
www.rascalscooters.com

Lark of America
800-558-7786
atyler@larkofamerica.com
www.larkofamerica.com

Palmer Industries
607-754-2957
800-847-1304
palmer@palmerind.com
www.palmerind.com

CCTVs

Enhanced Vision Systems
Developed the first voice-activated CCTV; also
specializes in portable models and low-vision
products. Call for a risk-free, no-pressure
demonstration from a representative near you.
800-440-9476
sales@enhancedvision.com
www.enhancedvision.com

Innoventions, Inc.
Well recognized for the Primer, a lightweight, inexpensive handheld camera that works with your computer or TV. Also sells the Magni-Cam and Triad. Will refer you to a local low-vision center or eye doctor for a demonstration; guarantees a free ten-day trial period after purchase.
800-854-6554
magnicam@magnicam.com
www.magnicam.com

MagniSight, Inc.
Owned and operated by people with low vision. Well recognized for the Explorer, which offers many good features, and for PC-compatible video magnifiers. Call for a risk-free, no-pressure demonstration from a representative near you.
800-753-4767
sales@magnisight.com
www.magnisight.com

Optelec
Optelec's products include the ClearView line, the Voyager Braille Display, and a wide range of handheld magnifiers.
800-828-1056
info@optelec.com
www.optelec.com

TeleSensory, Inc.
Well recognized for their Aladdin line, also offers
portable battery-operated units and the less
expensive Atlas camera unit, which plugs into
your monitor or TV. Call for a risk-free
demonstration from a local representative.
800-804-8004
info@telesensory.com
www.telesensory.com

COMPUTERS AND SOFTWARE

Ai Squared
Makers of ZoomText
802-362-3612
sales@aisquared.com
www.aisquared.com

Beyond Sight
Founded by Jim Misener, a blind businessman
from Denver. Provides advice and retails
computer-adaptive equipment, including high-
tech computers, speech synthesizers, and
coordinated and custom systems. Small selection
of other low-vision products.
303-795-6455
www.beyondsight.com

IBM
Maker of ViaVoice for Windows and Macintosh
888-ShopIBM (product code YEC98)

www-4.ibm.com/software/speech or www.ibm.com
(search term "ViaVoice")

Freedom Scientific (includes Henter-Joyce, Arkenstone, and Blazie Engineering)

Makers of MAGic, JAWS for Windows,
Arkenstone OPENbook, and Braille note takers
Blind/Low Vision Division
800-444-4443
www.freedomscientific.com
www.blazie.com

Innovative Rehabilitation Technologies, Inc. (IRTI)

IRTI specializes in retailing high-tech systems
for people with vision loss, four-track cassette
players, Arkenstone products, talking computers
and software, screen reading software, and
CCTVs.
800-322-4784
info@irti.net
www.irti.net

Kurzweil Educational Systems, Inc.

Makers of Kurzweil Scanners
800-894-5374
info@kurzweiledu.com
www.kurzweiledu.com

G. W. Micro, Inc.
Makers of Window-Eyes
260-489-3671
webmaster@gwmicro.com
www.gwmicro.com

PulseData/HumanWare
Makers of Braille hardware and software. Also retails other software products.
800-722-3393
www.humanware.com

Scansoft (includes Lernout & Hauspie and Dragon Systems)
Makers of Voice Xpress, Dragon Naturally Speaking
800-654-1187
800-380-1234
www.scansoft.com

APPENDIX D

Driving, Civil Rights, Tax Benefits, and Donations and Bequests

DRIVING

If you have low vision and would like to continue driving, read chapter 13 in this book, contact your state's DMV for their vision requirements, and consult with your optometrist or ophthalmologist. If you decide to try driving with a restricted license or using bioptic lenses (if they are permissible in your state), you may want to contact a driver rehabilitation specialist in your area for training on their use and for DMV driver's test coaching. To find a specialist, contact the Association for Driver Rehabilitation Specialists at 608-884-8833 or visit their Web site directory at www.driver-ed.org. You may also want to read a copy of Eli and Doron Peli's book, *Driving with Confidence: A Practical Guide to Driving with Low Vision* (River Edge, NJ: World Scientific Publishing, 2002), which provides tables of state vision requirements and driving regulations.

For general driving over fifty-five, the American Association of Retired Persons (AARP) offers a driver improvement course especially designed for seniors, the 55 Alive program. See their Web site at www.aarp.org/55alive or call 888-227-7669 for a class in your area.

Above all, if you are not eligible to drive, do not despair. Read all of chapter 13 and part II of this book for more information and alternatives.

CIVIL RIGHTS: YOUR ADA

The Americans with Disabilities Act (ADA) is a federal civil rights law passed in 1990. It protects people with low vision from discrimination by restaurants, stores, banks, public transportation, government offices, and employers. (This means, for example, that you cannot be denied equal service in a restaurant just because their menu print is too small to see.) While most people with macular degeneration do not encounter outright discrimination, if you feel you have been unfairly treated, you may want to remind the offender that you are protected by the ADA and find out whether it applies to your situation.

For complete information on your rights, see the Department of Justice Web site at www.usdoj.gov/crt/ada or call the Disability and Business Technical Assistance Center at 800-949-4232.

For complete information on your rights when traveling by air, including the rules for wheelchairs and walkers, visit the U.S. Department of Transportation Aviation Consumer Protection Division Web site at www.dot.gov/ airconsumer/pubs or write for a brochure from the Consumer Information Center, P.O. Box 100, Pueblo, CO 81009.

YOUR FEDERAL TAX BENEFITS

If you have less than 20/200 vision in your better eye, you are "legally blind" according to the U.S. government and you qualify for a special federal tax deduction that may be worth at least $1,000 and possibly more, depending on your age and marital status. Check with your tax adviser or the IRS for specific information on this year's tax benefits for the blind.

DONATIONS AND BEQUESTS: HOW TO MAKE SURE YOUR MONEY HELPS

One of the best ways to make a difference is to donate to research or public service organizations. Unfortunately, there are an increasing number of well-marketed but marginally legitimate "nonprofits" that aggressively solicit money for research into cures for macular degeneration and blindness or for community support. Most of this money goes to administrative expenses and shadow employees whose chief aim is to pocket your donations. They give relatively little to the research and services they claim to support. Here are a few tips for foiling the hucksters:

- Avoid contributing to groups that send you requests for money in the mail, especially if they use common scare tactics or promise cures for macular degeneration or blindness.

- Never donate any money based solely on a Web site, no matter how polished it seems. Call or E-mail for an annual report before you commit.

- Never donate a significant amount of money to any organization without reviewing their annual report and asking your attorney, your doctor, and the macular degeneration organizations listed in appendix A about their reputation.

- Nonprofits should never spend more than 50 percent of their funds on administration or other expenses. Avoid giving to organizations that do not meet this standard.

- Consider giving to a research program at a major university or an established medical facility or nonprofit visual rehabilitation program in your area, especially if you have enjoyed their services. Alternatively, choose a nationally respected organization such as the Foundation Fighting Blindness (for research) and the American Foundation for the Blind (for services and publications).

- Consider giving to one of the macular degeneration organizations listed in appendix A, especially if you are a member or have enjoyed their support (the authors receive no compensation for donations to organizations mentioned in this book).

Research Updates and Nutrition Studies

RESEARCH UPDATES

For current medical research and clinical trial information, contact the following organizations:

1. Call Macular Degeneration Partnership (MDP) toll-free at 888-430-9898 (press 1 on the main menu) for recorded monthly research updates, or visit their Web site at **www.amd.org**.

2. Join one or more of the national macular degeneration organizations and receive quarterly newsletters with research updates (see appendix A for contact information).

3. Visit the National Eye Institute (NEI) Web site at **www.nei.nih.gov**. The NEI is a division of the National Institutes of Health that funds major medical research in the United States.

4. Visit the Foundation Fighting Blindness (FFB) Web site at **www.blindness.org**. Updates are also available by regular mail or E-mail. The FFB is a nonprofit organization that funds major medical research in the United States.

NUTRITION STUDIES

The Age-Related Eye Disease Study Group. "A Randomized, Placebo-Controlled, Clinical Trial of High-Dose Supplementation with Vitamins C and E, Beta Carotene and Zinc for Age-Related Macular Degeneration and Vision Loss." *Archives of Ophthalmology* 119 (October 2001): 1417–36.

Heuberger, Roschelle A., Ph.D., Julie A. Mares-Perlman, Ph.D., Ronald Klein, M.D., Barbara E. K. Klein, M.D., Amy E. Millen, B.S., and Mari Palta, Ph.D. "Relationship of Dietary Fat to Age-Related Maculopathy in the Third National Health and Nutrition Examination Study." *Archives of Ophthalmology* 119 (December 2001): 1833–38.

Seddon, Johanna M., M.D., Bernard Rosner, Ph.D., Robert D. Sperduto, M.D., Lawrence Yannuzzi, M.D., Julia A. Haller, M.D., Norman P. Blair, M.D., and Walter Willett, M.D. "Dietary Fat and Risk for Advanced Age-Related Macular Degeneration." *Archives of Ophthalmology* 119 (August 2001): 1191–99.

Seddon, Johanna M., M.D., and the Eye Disease Case-Control Study Group. "Dietary Carotenoids, Vitamins A, C, and E, and Advanced Age-Related Macular Degeneration." *Journal of the AMA (JAMA)* 272, no. 8 (November 9, 1994): 1413–20.

Canada and Canadians
with AMD

Most of the resources listed in the previous appendixes are intended for Canadian readers, too. However, we know that some entries don't apply across the border, so we've included this appendix for our favorite neighbors. If you know of any other resources especially for Canadians that we should include in the next edition, please write to us about them at the contact address or E-mail listed on the "About the Authors" page that follows. Thank you!

FINDING A VISUAL REHABILITATION PROGRAM IN YOUR AREA

The Canadian National Institute for the Blind (CNIB)
CNIB provides a wide range of programs and resource referrals for people with vision loss throughout Canada, from Yellowknife, NT, to St. John's, NF. To find the service center nearest you, call the national office or visit the CNIB Web site and click on "Contact Us."

416-486-2500 (national office)
www.cnib.org

READING, WATCHING, AND LISTENING

Canadian National Institute for the Blind Library (CNIB Library)
CNIB's library offers a fantastic collection including 16,000 unabridged books on tape, eight popular magazines on tape, 15,000 Braille books and magazines, and more than 250 films and PBS programs on video with Descriptive Video Service (DVS). CNIB membership also includes a free four-track tape player on indefinite loan. You can also purchase a CNIB-compatible (often listed as "NLS" compatible; the NLS is the U.S. version of CNIB) player from the LS&S catalog listed in appendix C. Call for an application and information on other library programs.
416-480-7520 (Toronto)
800-268-8818 (nationwide in Canada)
library@lib.cnib.ca
www.cnib.ca

VoicePrint (National Broadcast Reading Service)
VoicePrint is Canada's twenty-four-hour audio newsstand. Every day, volunteers record full-length articles, columns, and feature reports

related to news and sports, health, entertainment, science, and more. Content is selected from more than 100 Canadian newspapers and magazines. VoicePrint is delivered via satellite, cable, and the Internet to 8.3 million homes throughout Canada. You can also listen to VoicePrint by tuning to the SAP channel of CBC Newsworld on your local cable TV station. Call or visit their Web site for programming and access information.
416-422-4222 (Toronto)
800-567-6755 (nationwide)
nbrs@nbrscanada.com
www.voiceprint.ca

DRIVING

Provincial governments tend to require 20/40 vision in your better eye for an unrestricted noncommercial driver's license, and the use of bioptic telescopes is rare, although this may be changing. For example, a 1999 Supreme Court case, *Terry Grismer* [estate] v. *British Columbia Council of Human Rights et al.*, successfully challenged the province's strict vision requirements for driving, which has resulted in new individual skill evaluations for drivers in British Columbia who do not meet the province's vision standards. For current rules, contact your province's Insurance Company or Department of Motor Vehicles. You'll find the number in the blue pages of your phone book. If you have been denied a license on the basis of your vision and you feel you are able to drive safely, you may want to contact your province's human rights council for information on appealing.

CIVIL RIGHTS

You are protected from some forms of discrimination on the basis of your vision by federal and provincial human rights acts and by the constitution's Charter of Rights and Freedoms. If you feel you have been treated unfairly by an employer, a public establishment, or a transportation provider, contact the following offices for more information: your province's Human Rights Council, your local CNIB office (see CNIB entry in "Reading, Watching, and Listening"), and the Canadian Federal Human Rights Council (call 800-622-6232).

TAXES

You may be eligible for a nonrefundable federal disability tax credit of $6,000 or more. To apply, you must file Form T2201, the Disability Tax Credit Certificate, with your income tax return. The form requires certification of disability from your eye doctor or family doctor. For eligibility questions and more information or to order forms in large print, on computer diskette or audiocassette, or in Braille, call 800-267-1267 weekdays during business hours (Eastern Time). There may also be opportunities for tax relief at the local and provincial level. Check with your municipality and provincial tax offices.

Index

A

ABCR gene, 97–98

activities in the community, 389–99

acuity and acuity measurements, 34–7.

See also driving

airlines and airplanes, 359–61.

See also travelling, 355–59

alternative or natural therapies.

See also nutrition and diet

  healing fruits, 124–27

  healing practices, 127–31

AMDATS: Age-Related Macular Degeneration and Thalidomide Study, 64–5

Americans with Disabilities Act, 430–31

Amsler grid, 46–51

Anacortave Acetate, 80

angiograms, 56–59

antiangiogenics, 76–80

antioxidants and free radicals, 93–95.

See also nutrition and diet

apheresis (rheotherapy), 74–5

AREDS: Age Related Eye Disease Study, 115

asking others for help or assistance, 213–14.

See also visual rehabilitation

Associations for people with AMD, 195–97, 403–04

audio-books. See listening

free radicals and antioxidants, 93–95.
    See also nutrition and diet
friends, tips for 225–235

G
gas bubble treatment, 59–60
genetics of AMD, 89–93, 96–98
geographic atrophy, 20
ginko biloba, 118
glare, 162, 265–67, 273–74
glaucoma, 39–40
greens (leafy green vegetables), 104–107, 132–36
    recipes for, 137–51

H
hallucinations, 236–52
hereditary factors, 89–90, 96–98
hypertension as a risk factor, 28–29
holistic treatments. *See* natural or alternative
    therapies
home adaptations, 267–74, 362–87
humor, keeping a sense of, 211–12.
    See also stories of people with AMD

I
ICG: indocyanine green angiogam, 57–58
imaginary images (Charles Bonnet Syndome),
    236–52
Interferon, 64–65
Internet communities, 196–97, 407–408
invisibility of vision loss with AMD, see "It's

invisibility of vision loss with AMD *(cont'd)*
Hard to See If It Isn't Happening to You,"
158–59

J
joining a support group or AMD organization,
194–202

K
kale, 104–107, 132–36,
recipes, 137–51

L
lamps, 269–73
large print
books. *See* Reading Workshop
checks, 375–76
products (phones, calendars, recipes books).
See product catalogs, 422–423
laser, laser photocoagulation, 43–46, 52–59
experimental laser 67–69
legal blindness and blindness, 31–38
letter recognition, 289–94. *See also* Reading
Workshop
Library of Congress Talking Book Program,
416–17. *See also* listening
lighting and light bulbs, 264–75 (chapter 10)
at home, 266–272
in public places, 274–75
light sensitivity (glare), 162, 265–67, 273–74

recognizing faces, see "Contrast Sensitivity,"
160–62
rehabilitation. *See* visual rehabilitation
research process and progress, 62–64. *See also*
clinical trials, 65–66
research updates, 42–43, 434
restaurants and dining out, 204–205, 274–75,
393–94
retina, 15–19
rheo-therapy, 74–75
rhuFabV2, 80
ride-sharing, 350–51
risk factors for AMD, 27–29, 86–90
rod and cone cells, 16–17
RPE: retinal pigment epithelium, 18–19

S
salmon and sardines, *see* fish and fish oil,
109–114, 124
salmon recipe, 148, sardine recipe, 144
scooters, 349–50, 423–24
scotoma (blind spot). *See also* stories of people
with AMD
from laser treatment, 52–56
from wet and dry AMD, 10–11, 26
maximizing your vision with it, 282–89
seeing things that aren't there, 236–52
selenium, 115–116, 124
shock of AMD, 164–67, 173–74
shopping, 391–92
smoking, 27, 90, 100–101

Index

smoking (*cont'd*)
  smoking and beta-carotene, 116, 119
software. *See* computer software
spinach, 104–07, 132–136,
  recipes, 137–51
"Spinach that Sees," 82
SST: Submacular Surgery Trials, 70
Stargardt's disease, 97–98, 196
stem cells, 73
St. John's Wort, 192
stories about ourselves 202–211
stories of people with AMD. *See also* memoirs,
    194–95, 408–09
  authors' family, 1–6
  Bixley Bennet, *see* "Live Through Reaching
    Out, 222
  Dolly Kowalksi and Joe Toscano, *see* "It's Hard
    To See If," 158–159
  Evangeline, *see* "Live Through Faith," 223–24
  Georgette, *see* "Live Through Love," 220–21
  Grace Olsen, 165–69, with Lily, see "Be Honest
    with Friends," 214–215
  Jack, *see* "The Power of Positive Stories,"
    207–210
  Linda Olsen, 198–99
  Natalie Steele, *see* "The Blindness Story," 204–06
  Pat Reynolds, *see* "The Macular Degeneration
    Slide," 206–07
  Rosa Garcia, *see* "The Stories We Tell About
    Ourselves," 203–04
  Sam Weinberg, 178–81, 236–37

451

vegetables *(cont'd)*
  recipes 137–151
VEGF: Vascular Endothelial Growth Factor,
  76–77
verteporfin. *see* Visudyne
veterans and Veterans Administration (VA), 406
VIM study: Visudyne In Minimally Classic CNV,
  55
vision. *See also* low vision, visual rehabilitation
  aids. *See* magnifiers, computers, talking
    products
  and driving. *See* driving
  blind spot. *See* scotoma
  detecting changes in, *see* Amsler grid, 46–51
  experience of AMD, *see* "So What Can You
    See?" 159–63
  monitoring your, *see* Amsler grid, 46–51
  peripheral, *see* "AMD affects only the Macula,"
    30–34
  phantom (Charles Bonnet Syndrome), 236–52
  vocabulary and definitions, 34–38
visual aids. *See* magnifiers, computers, talking
    products
visual rehabilitation. *See* Part III of the book for
    a complete home program
  definition of, introduction to, 171–172, 255–63
  experience with. *See* stories of people with AMD
  depression, 187–94
  family and friends participating, 233–34
  finding a program in your area, 257–58,
    405–407

About the Authors

LYLAS G. MOGK, M.D., is the founding director of the Visual Rehabilitation and Research Center of Michigan, part of Henry Ford Health System Eye Care Services. Dr. Mogk is the chair of the American Academy of Ophthalmology Vision Rehabilitation Committee and speaks regularly to physicians, occupational therapists, and community organizations nationwide about macular degeneration and visual rehabilitation. She lives with her husband, John, and her father, Charles R. Good, who has advanced AMD. Despite his severe vision loss, Dr. Mogk's father lives a full and active life following the visual rehabilitation program in this book.

MARJA MOGK, is completing a doctorate from the University of California at Berkeley. Her dissertation, *Narrating Vision: Disability, Aging, and Autobiography,* focuses on oral and written accounts of living with vision loss by older and younger adults. She is Lylas and John Mogk's daughter.

CONTACT US

We truly hope this book is an important resource for everyone with macular degeneration or at risk for it. If you would like to share a tip for living with low vision, a story or anecdote, or a recipe for our next edition or if you have comments on this edition, please write to us care of Lylas G. Mogk, M.D., at 15401 E. Jefferson Avenue, Grosse Pointe, MI 48230. Take care and best wishes.